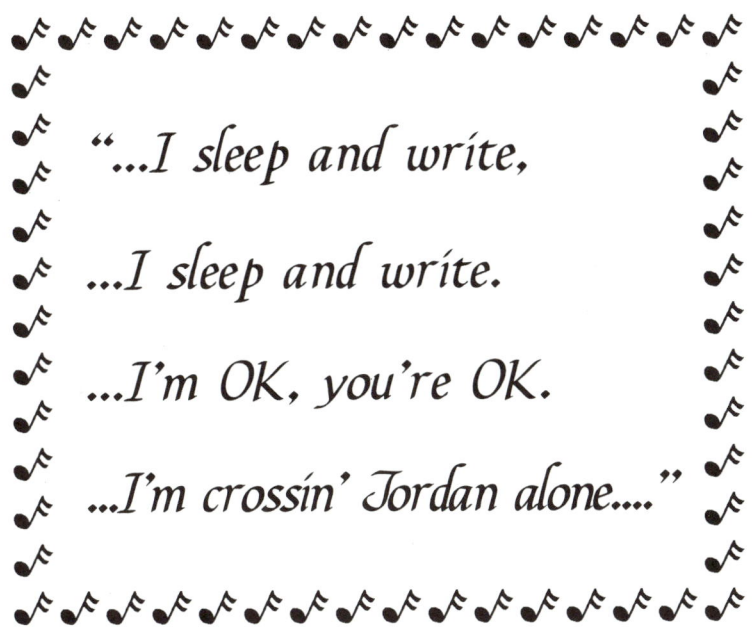

Eunice's final journal entry

on January 10, 1994.

Eunice
She Loved Life

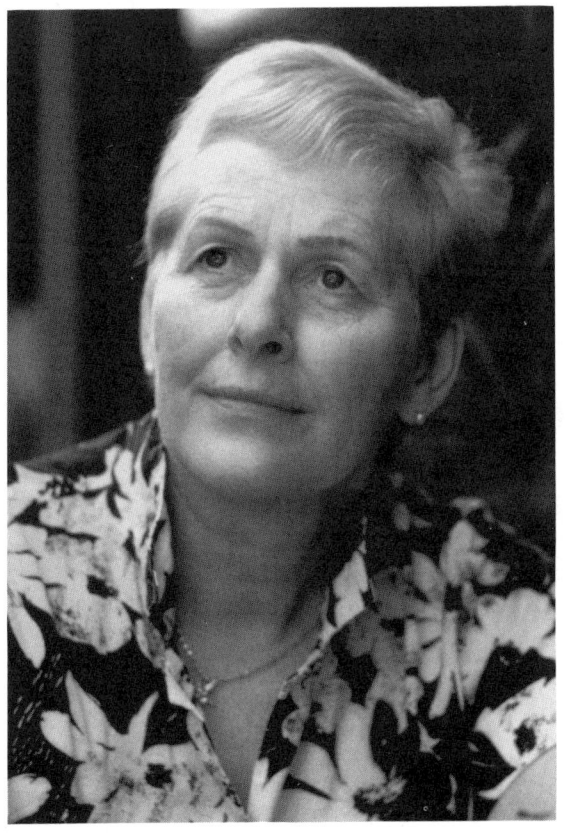

Photo by Susan Urban

"COME THEN, MY LOVE, COME. FOR SEE THE WINTER
IS PAST....THE RAINS ARE OVER AND GONE.
THE FLOWERS APPEAR ON THE EARTH
AND THE DOVE IS HEARD AGAIN IN OUR LAND.
ARISE, MY LOVE, AND COME TO ME."

- SONG OF SONGS

Eunice—She Loved Life

Copyright © 1996
by
Masthof Press

*Photo collages by Sylvia Francois and Marge Edwards.
Sketch on back cover by Peter Mast.
Cover designed by Marshall's Graphics.*

Library of Congress Number: 96-94110
International Standard Book Number: 1-883294-35-5

Published by
Masthof Press
*Route 1, Box 20
Morgantown, PA 19543*

DEDICATED TO THE CHILDREN

Wendell Dean
Colleen Joy
Timothy Brent
Jill Sue
Peter Henry
Hans Anton

"...the timeless in you
is aware of life's timelessness
and knows that
yesterday is but today's memory and
tomorrow is today's dream
and that which sings and contemplates in you
is still dwelling
within the bounds of that moment
which scattered the stars into space...."

- *Kahlil Gibran*

ACKNOWLEDGEMENTS

Writing about Eunice, my wife for forty-one years, would not have been an impossible task in itself, but to communicate her soul and the emotions that peaked during the last three years of her life was monumental. Her determination in writing the journal, difficult as it was, allows us to empathize with and understand this special woman.

Many people played a part in presenting the book. Our daughter, Colleen, encouraged me to bring Eunice's diaries to the public and helped in some of the proofreading.

Phee Sherline, a friend of the family who lives in California, said, "Your story is bigger than life. Why don't you write a book?" She helped edit the manuscript and offered suggestions in its design.

John Ruth, Eunice's brother from Pennsylvania, has always been our inspiration to write. He offered to read the manuscript and to give suggestions.

Sylvia Francois, a friend from Woodstock area, offered to arrange the collage displays of Eunice's life.

Susan Urban, a professional photographer and singer from Chicago, provided the picture of Eunice and me.

Eunice's sister, Martyne and husband Conrad Wetzel, read the material and helped me through the emotional strain of making this book possible.

Other friends from the Woodstock community read all or parts of the manuscript and have been my constant support: My son Hans and wife Sherry who live nearby always welcome me home; neighbor Letty Harting; John and Esther Hackman, our closest friends over many years; Steve and Sylvia Francois have carried the most responsibility for the Singalong; and the MASTHOUSE committee for its commitment to keep the Saturday night music event flowing.

My son Dean gave me space in his California home to do much of the final work on his computer and to coach me in computer language and design. My other children in California, Jill, Peter, Tim and wife Holly, have been my link to Eunice through the winter months.

*- Don Mast
March 1996*

PREFACE

Eunice's story of her struggle with cancer the last three years of her life may not be much different emotionally from other cancer victims. This is her story, a kind of love story of a woman who believed that:

> "...love is patient and kind;
> love is not jealous or boastful;
> it is not arrogant or rude.
> Love does not insist on its own way;
> it is not irritable or resentful;
> it does not rejoice at wrong but rejoices in the right.
> Love bears all things, believes all things,
> hopes all things, endures all things...."

Our love for each other and our children was woven around the complexities of religious mores, parenthood, justice, community, economics, alcohol, differing lifestyles and geographic mobility, and finally cancer, but always there was music and friends. The irony for Eunice is that she had no family history of cancer. Except for her love for chocolates, she was extremely health-conscious. She was the epitome of a bright and positive person who loved life and laughed often. Prior to the diagnosis I do not ever remember her being depressed.

During the last six months of her life, Eunice regularly wrote her thoughts which form the basis for this book. The regular type print are her words taken almost verbatim, while the italicized parts are my own explanations and details of her flashbacks to a previous time in her life. The letters are representative of the many people who wrote expressing their feelings toward Eunice. The quotes are inspirational reminders to look at our lives with positive perspectives. Her medical history at the end will be helpful for those who try to make some sense out of the mystery of the existence of cancer. The article from the Chicago Tribune *will help explain the creation by Eunice of an eclectic gathering place for people to hear music and to find community.*

The names that appear are real people who provided real help, a community of love. For those of you who may never have met Eunice, I hope you will feel her unique spirit from the openness with which she wrote her daily thoughts that has enabled her children, friends, and me to deal with death as just another facet of life. Her God was real and compassionate. Never during her illness did Eunice or I blame God for such a human tragedy as cancer. Her expectancy of the new journey beyond death is spiritually rewarding.

- Don Mast
March 1996

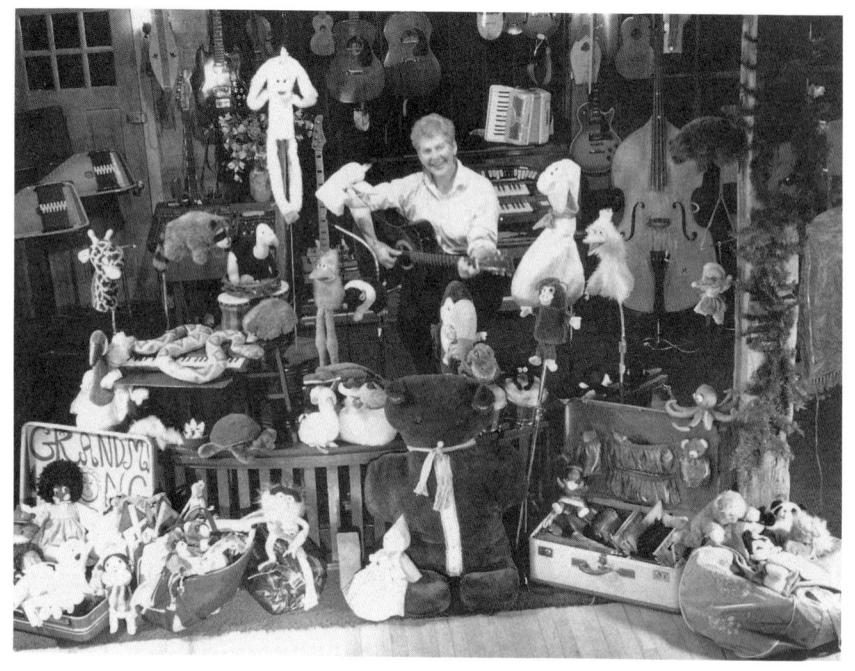

Photo by Sylvia Francois

Eunice with her puppets and instruments on the Masthouse stage.

x

EUNICE—She Loved Life

Memorial Day, 1993: It's 10 o'clock...time for Channel 7 News. Don and I are in bed; he's sleeping and every once in awhile I poke him and tell him he needs to change his position to stop his snoring! He usually jerks awake and asks, "Was I really snoring?"

"Yes, one of these nights I'll tape record it and prove it to you."

I must do that some day.

Three years have passed since Eunice wrote these words. Even now I stare at the diary in disbelief that she is no longer here to revitalize my spirit and share my life.

I just finished watching the special on Bill Monroe. He fascinates me, as do many performers. I identify, in a way, with them and have a craving in my soul to make music, all kinds of music. That is one of the things I feel so grateful for tonight...the joy of music, a gift from God. It has made our lives rich. I've been real blessed. What a wonderful life I've had! So many neat people have touched my life. What a wonderful home with caring parents, Henry and Susan Ruth of Harleysville, Pennsylvania, who faithfully took me to Finland Mennonite Church and instilled God's love in me. That is still my favorite Bible message: "God is love." It says it all. It helps me decide priorities. I want to be faithful to show God's love in every situation in life.

I feel so strongly that "To whom much is given, much is required." I want to give back. I feel there is a reason we're here on this earth, and it's not just to get all we can. I've learned long ago that "Love is something if you give it away, you'll end up having more," a song by Malvina Reynolds, whom I have greatly admired. She was a white-haired grandma from New York who couldn't sing well but wrote a lot of meaningful songs.

THE MAGIC PENNY

It's just like a magic penny,
Hold it tight and you won't have any;
Lend it, spend it and you'll have so many
They'll roll all over the floor....

Money's dandy and we like to use it,
But love is better if you don't refuse it;
It's a treasure and you'll never lose it
Unless you lock up your door....

Love is something if you give it away,
Give it away, give it away, give it away;
Oh love is something if you give it away,
You'll end up having more.

What a miracle that my parents sent me to Lancaster Mennonite High School, fifty miles west of Philadelphia, where I met Donny Mast the first day down by the Mill Stream where a small group was playing a get-acquainted game. Don was a very popular junior and I, a 14-year-old shy freshman. When his cousin, Ada Ruth, came up to me and said, "Donny Mast likes you," I was positive (I still tease Don to this day) that he was just interested in me because of my famous brother John or my popular sister Lois. Much later he told me the real reason he was attracted to me...and I won't tell you why!

It will be a secret no longer that Eunice was a beautiful young girl, desired by many sixteen-year-old boys, and teasingly shy. A boarding school for Mennonites was indeed a rarity in the 1940's and we all felt privileged to be given this opportunity by our parents for a private high school education. During those years the students numbered approximately 200, half of whom were dormitory residents.

Don and I spent our free time playing ping-pong. He was the school champ. I was always picked first on his ball team, although not because of my skill. I was so painfully shy that I would run the other way if I saw him coming down the sidewalk toward me. My friend Erma, whose boyfriend—Harold Rohrer—was Don's best friend, helped take care of my shyness by planning activities such as tennis and skating on the Mill Stream (the only activity where holding hands with Don was allowed). One time during skating, a friend and I broke through the ice, managed to get to shore, and after a change of clothes, got to chapel late, which was a sin. Don was the song leader and, in seeing us arrive late, was distracted and gave the wrong pitch to start the song.

In 1947 during my sophomore year a simply awful thing happened! Sister Kaufman, the girls' matron, an "old maid" in the true sense of the word, intruded into my life. She was not very personable, a kind of busybody. She decided that Don and I were becoming too friendly; consequently, she wrote a letter to my parents requesting that they put an end to our relationship.

Sister Kaufman had been so impressed with John and Lois, my siblings, and she had wanted to protect me from the likes of Donny Mast, this wild boy from a "lower" spiritual family than mine. When Mom informed me that I could no longer see Donny, I was livid. Mom was the one who related to the kids; Pop listened quietly from the living room during family discussions which usually took place around the kitchen table. He would express his opinions later to Mom which then filtered down to us. It was not easy to explain to Don what had transpired, but we decided that time would heal; we'd soon begin writing again.

A few years later in the spring of 1950, my brother John explained to Mom that Donny seemed to be a spiritual fellow while a student at Eastern Mennonite College in Harrisonburg, Virginia. With that bit of encouragement, Mom allowed me to pursue my relationship with Donny again. So what do I do now? I called my friend Erma who helped us get back together. I thanked God many times because Donny Mast is the best!

Family values were strong for Eunice. There was a respect for what your parents said, a fear of Pop, as well as a fire and brimstone theology that diminished the temptation to stray. Eunice's mother, in particular, kept communications open with all the children. The fact that they would spend the money to send all their five children fifty miles to a Christian boarding school was evidence of their dedication and belief in a strong Christian education.

The years 1950 to the summer of 1952 Eunice and I communicated by mail. She graduated from the Mennonite high school in Harrisonburg, Virginia, in 1951 and I attended the same institution as a college freshman in 1951-52. Somehow we still managed to make wedding plans for September 6, 1952, even though Eunice claimed I never really proposed to her...and I have a memory lapse.

We were married on the home farm in Chester County, Pennsylvania, the farm where Don was born and where his father and grandfather before him lived. Imagine my excitement to learn that I would be the queen in this huge ten-room house after growing up in a house that could fit into three rooms of this one. Don's dad said we could have this 150-acre farm. I was tickled pink, even with all the decorating we had to do, using wild wallpaper (ask Jill to see the samples), and furnishing it with all new furniture including a new piano.

So the wedding day arrived with 200 people invited. Don's mother and helpers prepared a full Mennonite meal with all the trimmings. How unusual to see some of Don's Amish relatives arrive by horse and buggy. Don and I had decided to sing a duet together, a part of the cantata "David the Shepherd Boy" by George Root, taken from the story of David and Jonathan in the Bible. (We revised it for a man and woman.) During practice, I always ended up crying so Don's brother, Ike, stepped in and sang it with Don at the last minute:

> "Since first my soul was knit to thine
>   I have been true to thee;
> My heart is thine, thy heart is mine,
>   And shall forever be.
> I go not from thee when I go
>   And come not when I come;
> Whatever lot is mine to know
>   With thee is rest and home."

My brother John married us and Martyne, my sister, played "Bless This House" on the piano. Then we were off to the Pocono Mountains for a honeymoon. Don's mother made sure we had enough food for our week in a cabin...potatoes, canned beef, chicken, etc. I didn't yet know how to cook; you'll have to ask my mother why. I was the hired girl growing up on the farm so I milked the cows and Lois did the easy housework. I was quite skilled at squirting milk from a cow's teat directly into the mouths of our family of cats that always were present at milking time. Also, I was the designated washer of the milking buckets, using high-powered B-K solution. I've often wondered whether that cleaning powder was the cause of my cancer.

Home from the honeymoon and time to get down to some hard farm and housework. My memory of cabbage harvesting includes a scary truck ride to the field with me holding a sharp knife used in cutting off the head. The truck went around a turn and I fell out clutching the knife in my hand. I didn't even receive a bruise...with Dean about five months old in my stomach. Dean, our first child, was born August 10, 1953, a difficult birth at 9 lbs. 3 oz. I cannot recall any worse pain in my life....I wanted to die!

Don's folks lived on the edge of the farm in a house newly-built by Don's dad. Usually his dad would arrive at the barn early in the morning before Don got out of bed, and I felt guilty that here we were given the farm and now his dad was doing a lot of the work. Don's mother taught me to do canning and gardening. We even butchered our own livestock.

Eunice was two weeks from nineteen and I was twenty as we attempted to learn the roles of a husband and wife. We wanted to prove Dad's confidence in us in running the farm. We were active members of the Maple Grove Mennonite Church in Atglen. Although Eunice was a transplant in this community, she was loved. There were new mores to get adjusted to for Eunice, as she explains later. One "sin" we agreed needed to be reckoned with was the game of cards. One evening with penitent hearts, we went down to the basement of our farmhouse, opened the door of the coal furnace, and watched our deck of cards go up in smoke. We felt a sense of pride in our religiosity and were content. Both of us grew up in church communities with strict moral codes against drinking, smoking, swearing, and going to movies, but the Bible, God, and the church helped sustain strong family ties. I can't remember any divorces in our community of 400 church members.

Two years passed. Farming took more of my time than I thought it would. We had no intention of dissolving our involvement with our friends who lived in Lancaster, twenty miles away. We soon learned, though, we couldn't put in a full day's work on the farm and then run around at night.

It was I rather than Eunice who first thought of moving. She was in love with the place, but she also wanted me to be happy. In June of 1954, after nearly two years of farming, we filled a truck with our belongings, leaving behind a beautiful farm to my older brother, Ike, and moved to western Pennsylvania near Pittsburgh to our second home.

Don was employed as the secretary to the sales manager of our Mennonite Publishing House in Scottdale. With us was our nine-month-old Dean. This move to Scottdale was a Godsend. We worked among respected leaders of the Mennonite Church, whom we knew only by reading their articles in our church magazines. We were so impressed by their warm welcome in helping us find a place to live. Temporarily we stayed in the guest quarters of Ralph and Liz Hernley. They helped Don and me sort through some of the cultural baggage I had brought along from a much more conservative community in the East. Through tears and talking I finally believed maybe it wasn't wrong to wear shoes with the toes out or to pray without a prayer veiling, etc.

I believed I was hearing new truths. After all, these were respected church leaders. On December 9, 1954, Colleen was born, an easy birth in comparison. We loved our little family and soon fit into the community and church life.

During that year in Scottdale I became more aware of my need to complete my college education to pursue a professional teaching career. Consequently, in June 1955, we moved, again, to Harrisonburg, Virginia. Eastern Mennonite College felt like home to us because this is where Eunice had graduated from high school only four years prior, and I had attended my first year of college in 1952. We built on our friendships with former students. I had to find a job while going to school and trying to be a husband and father.

The spring of 1956 brought two new challenges. Our third child, Timothy Brent, was born in March and Don's mother died of cancer in April. This meant three diaper babies under three years old; now I was getting concerned how to stop this pattern that with each new move we were rewarded with a baby. But each one was such a joy that we only considered ourselves lucky. Of course, there was no such thing as "Pampers," but Don dutifully helped wash out the diapers. Towards the end of the school year Don's first cousin, Vic Stoltzfus who lived and went to college in Goshen, Indiana, persuaded us to move to Goshen where Don could complete his education in a more progressive setting.

Vic and Marie had been close to us through the years and we were enticed by what Vic described as a small group of college and seminary faculty/students who were revolutionizing the concept of the church. Well, we certainly didn't want to miss a new challenge, and there was no doubt we were experienced movers, so off we went, a little bit concerned whether this would mean a fourth child. We sold most of what we could easily part with, packed the rest in a U-Haul in back of our '53 Chevy, nestled the three kids into the car, and off we went over the Appalachian Mountains to the Midwest and to new surprises. From that summer of 1956 to Don's graduation in 1958 with a B.S. in Secondary Education there would be enough material for a book.

The nutshell version is that again our eyes were opened and our vision expanded beyond belief. Don's dad had divested himself of his excess funds to the six children which gave us enough to pay off college bills and buy a simple house in Goshen for $7,000. We loved the small college town and the comradeship of new friends and the joy of three kids who were getting accustomed to their nomadic parents. We soon discovered this Mennonite community had fewer taboos and that some church members actually went to movies. We reasoned that our new liberal education should include a sample of this vice, so with our friends' recommendation we asked Vic and Marie to baby-sit for us and we went to the theater to see *Friendly Persuasion*. Undoubtedly, there were love scenes in the movie that must have caused our passions to soar, but I can't remember feeling pangs of guilt.

The Goshen years directed our lives. This bastion of Mennonite theology and education was the right stimulus for us. The small group that Vic had used to bribe us into moving to Goshen was a collection of visionaries who believed that the church should be more than a place to go once a week. They were seminary professors/college teachers and wives, and a few starry-eyed college kids who appeared to be serious activists and we wanted to be in on the action. The ultimate outcome of these gatherings during 1956 and 1957 was the formation of a communal group which would attempt to "live" the gospel wherever that might lead. Eunice never could endure the endless meetings. She wanted to be a part but was more interested in serving the food and lighting the candles. During the spring of 1957 our little group decided to locate in a large city, which became Evanston, Illinois. There we would try to see whether a communal church could exist in an urban setting. After I graduated in 1958 we sold our Goshen house, shared the proceeds with the community in Evanston, and moved in with two other families at 727 Reba Place.

Those early years of Reba Place Fellowship (the name derived from the street on which the first two houses were located) have been the subject of many magazine articles, including a spot in *Time* magazine. Don and I were excited. This little farm girl was thrown into the big city.

Indeed, Eunice fit beautifully into this new life because she felt her faith was lived. She exuded confidence. Her creativity enriched all of those she met, both within the communal group as well as her daily contacts in the neighborhood. Mrs. Tedesco, who lived in the apartment next door, admired Eunice. This was a seventy-year-old lady who spoke glowingly of her years of working as a maid for Dr. Freud in Vienna. We used the name of her son, Hans, for our sixth child.

When I think of all the exciting times we've had at Eastern Mennonite College, the Publishing House, and Goshen and the wonderful friends we've had throughout all those moves, I feel so grateful; and always there was music...all kinds of music. The whole Reba Place experience was so good for us. We learned so much about ourselves, about God, about sharing and caring, about having fun, about money, and, yes, about music. Don gave me Thursday night out. In 1960 I decided to enroll at Old Town School of Folk Music and learn what I could. Don and I loved music all of our lives, but our vision was somewhat limited to church music. We had been weaned on hymns and didn't stray far from that until my introduction to "folk music" in Chicago. Don stayed home with our six children and off I went with a friend to this exciting school to learn to play the guitar.

> **"The universe is made of stories, not of atoms."**
> - *Muriel Rukeyser*

Actually Don had bought a ukulele for me at a garage sale months before and that just whetted my appetite for the real thing. After an audition by the dean of the school, Ray Tate, I was put in his advanced class...what a challenge! I would get home after midnight and still practice for hours so I wouldn't forget what I learned. I soon acquired a group of students from the commune and community who wanted to learn what I had been taught. It wasn't long before I was using my elementary guitar skills in our Sunday church meetings. The south side of Evanston where we lived had a growing number of Japanese families. The Murakami family, in particular, we learned to know through our son, Tim, who became friends with their twin sons, Kosei and Gensei.

Because of that friendship, there developed a group of seven Japanese mothers who persuaded me to teach them guitar; I didn't know Japanese and they knew no English, but we had a hilarious time in spite of it. "Mushi, Mushi" was our closest attempt at communication.

One "O Henry-type" story growing out of this friendship bears repeating. On the first Christmas following our acquaintance with the Murakamis, they invited us to their house for dinner and gifts. Eunice and I are very simple in our wardrobes...living on welfare standards, we had little choice...so we didn't know much about expensive jewelry or clothes much less own them. However, our Japanese friends weren't aware of our shortcomings and they presented us with pearls—Eunice was given a pin for her "thrift shop" dress and for me a tie-pin for a man who wears no ties. Being ignorant of and unaccustomed to jewelry due to our Mennonite "plain" upbringing, these gifts presented us with a dilemma...we weren't going to use these beautiful pieces. One custom of the Fellowship was to give each other a gift on "Three Kings Day." What better idea, Eunice thought, than to give one of the young girls this beautiful pin since Eunice wouldn't be using it anyway. As luck would have it, at a later date Mrs. Murakami asked Eunice why she didn't wear the pin with her dress. By some clever chicanery Eunice was able to retrieve the pin with the pearl and the story had a happy ending. I still have the pin which I never use, and Eunice's pin has since disappeared.

Anyway, I was determined that our children would appreciate the joys of making music. I was probably too pushy at times, but Don kept the balance with his casual attitude about not forcing music...to my frustration sometimes...but now he says I was right. Tim, Peter, and Hans play guitar well and the others enjoy music, so my time wasn't wasted. The years at the Evanston commune were the years of my greatest spiritual development.

"She blossomed where she was planted."

Although Don and I were raised in Mennonite homes in eastern Pennsylvania, most of our married life was lived on the fringes of the established church. The Reba Place Fellowship which eventually was enfranchised into the Mennonite fold was initially considered a "black sheep." We had always felt our involvement with causes enriched our spiritual lives. Our parents felt otherwise because we were not traditional Mennonites.

Our communal experiment predated the "Hippie" movement and, furthermore, had a Christian foundation. For us in the late 1950's there were few intentional communities on which to base our life together. We had some conversations and visits involving the Hutterites of the East Coast and of Canada. Now, thirty-five years later, this little fledgling community in Evanston, Illinois, is still alive and well, and continues to be a source of inspiration and healing to many people. Our children had many good adult role models who loved and cared for them.

The communal life brought us into contact with other like-minded movements eventually. One such community was Koinonia, an integrated rural group of families near Americus, Georgia. Their leader, Clarence Jordan, a southern Baptist, had a degree in agriculture and was a seminary graduate, plus he was a powerful speaker with an articulate southern drawl, a spell-binding story teller, and a writer. His *Cotton Patch Version of the Gospels* was adapted to drama and music by Harry Chapin. Don and I loved visiting them, and on one occasion experienced the hostilities of the KKK who appeared at night dressed in white hoods. They were respected mayors and school board members from the local towns who hated the efforts of Koinonia to eat and work with blacks in developing a pecan business. They came with guns and shot holes into the buildings.

Because of fierce hostilities, Koinonia had to adapt their pecan business to a mail order operation. Another effort that we watched them develop was building affordable housing for blacks on their property. I can remember meeting Millard Fuller, a twentish millionaire from New York who wanted to put his money and energy into something worthwhile. He saw the sprouting of new homes for the poor and helped turn the idea into the present internationally-known "Habitat for Humanity."

Since Reba Place was located in an integrated part of southern Evanston, Illinois, we were faced immediately with taking positions on open housing, school busing, and other issues related to the civil rights movement.

We did not consider our activist behaviors as a sign of debunking the "faith of our fathers." Rather, we felt the civil rights marches in Washington, voter registration in the South, anti-war demonstrations, sharing our money were a natural result of "living the gospel."

"Life is like music, it must be composed
by ear, feeling, and instinct, not by rule."
- *Samuel Butler*

The summer of 1959 brought another change in the life of our family. We heard from a friend of the Fellowship that many children were left abandoned in Korea due to the war. Through the Holt Agency in Oregon who had representatives in Seoul, we learned the procedure to adopt. We inquired into the possibilities of getting an older child because of our own younger children. However, during the next several months we received a call that there was a nine-month-old child abandoned who needed a home. So we agreed to take the younger child. By January 1960, we became aware that Eunice was pregnant again, but we were satisfied to know that Jill Sue would be arriving shortly and we could make the proper adjustment. As it turned out, there were delays in the adoption red-tape, and Jill arrived in Portland three weeks before Peter was born. Consequently, Eunice did not fly with me to Portland to meet Jill who by July 3rd was one and a half years old. By the time Peter arrived on July 27th we had moved into the first floor of the second Fellowship house at 714 Reba Place. This large Victorian building was adequate for us. We made generous use of the basement and various huge closets, one of which became the bedtime quarters of our sixth child, Hans, in November of 1962. We thought we had just about used up our need for new challenges until a new one appeared in May of 1964.

In 1964 a dentist from Dwight, Illinois, offered his twenty-room Catholic mission house in Campus, Illinois, to Reba Place to be used for retreats from the big city. It seemed ideal. Someone, however, needed to move there to set up the project. Of course, Don and I always seemed ready for a challenge, so we agreed with the Fellowship to spend a year in this small town of 200 Irish Catholics and be hosts to groups from Chicago. It didn't take long to pack our few belongings and convince our six kids to prepare for a long camping experience.

We were certainly naive about the effect on the local community when "big city kids," blacks in particular, would descend on this little "lily-white" town. This was the year of Malcolm X assassination and one year after President Kennedy's similar fate.

Don easily got a teaching job in Saunemin High School, sixteen miles away, and I tried to fit into the community with my charming children, and good will. Our immediate neighbors, the Foleys and their two children, were our greatest friends from the start. Almost nightly we went over to their house, played pinochle, and ate Tina's freshly baked sweet rolls.

The year was filled with startling events. The black youths were not at all discreet about making themselves known as they walked around town on these occasional weekends. One evening as we were enjoying the company of my sister, Martyne and Conrad, we heard a knock on the door about midnight. It was the sheriff of the town who was noticeably intoxicated. He warned us that if we continue to bring those "niggers" into town, someone would burn the house down, and to emphasize his point he marked a big "X" on the framework of the door with a piece of chalk. On another occasion our guests' car tires were slashed. We knew then what it was like being a minority.

(In the summer of 1965 after we had returned to Evanston, we learned that the sheriff's threat was carried out and the building was torched.)

One day when I walked across the lawn to visit the Foleys, I noticed Tina was crying when I came in the back door.

"What's wrong?" I asked.

"Didn't you see who just left by the front door?" Tina said. I glanced out the window and noticed Father Mooney, the local parish priest walking away.

"He doesn't want my kids to play with yours," she added. "But I gave him a piece of my mind!"

I tried to soothe the waters, but I couldn't wait to tell Don what had happened. We had been accustomed to more subtle discrimination in Evanston, but not quite this blatant. My mind went back to the comfortable life in our protected Mennonite communities of Goshen,

Virginia, and Pennsylvania; and I felt like a transplanted flower without proper nourishment.

Well, that evening when Don heard about it, he got up from the table and marched right over to Father Mooney's house and knocked on the parish door. We'd always been greeted with such pleasantries by him that I was shocked by the turn of events. According to Don, he asked Father Mooney for a Bible. Don then read to him a verse in Matthew 18.

"In Matthew," Don said, "we are told to speak to each other about our differences. Aren't two children of the same father, brothers?" The symbolism of Mennonites and Catholics being brothers united under God, I'm sure, was a novel concept to Father Mooney.

I doubt if anyone had confronted Father Mooney in this way before. He disputed everything Don told him about the rumors we had heard. In fact, at a later date he even asked us to play recorders at their Christmas mass, which we did.

Eunice was enjoying the life in Campus, Illinois, but it was not all easy for her. How those visitors loved her homemade bread and cooking, but there was strain. She suffered through a temporary illness that could never be identified. In spite of it, she exhibited an uncanny resiliency to difficult situations.

"The heart carries the feet."
- Hebrew Proverb

Eunice and I experienced another growth spurt during that year of separation from our fellow-church members at

Reba Place, and we were eager to see them again. Our 714 Reba Place house was waiting for us. Other Fellowship members who had been living there temporarily squeezed into smaller units. By the summer of 1965 the Fellowship had owned several large Victorian houses which the members were skillful enough to remodel so that several families could live in one house. Our location was only blocks from Lake Michigan, and Eunice and I would often take the kids on a hike to the beach. On one hot summer day, the beach was so crowded we lost five-year-old Peter. The lifeguard ordered everyone out of the water and a search began. It took us ten minutes to realize that Peter had walked the seven blocks home without telling us.

During the fall of 1969, Don and I began inviting people to our place for a "Hootenanny." The basement took on the appearance of a coffee house with spool tables, candles, and chess and checker sets. In less than a year, we outgrew the basement, and the Fellowship assisted in converting our four-car garage into additional space. The Vietnam War and the growing unrest with the civil rights movement gave impetus to many protest and peace songs. We were developing our musical skills and another dream was realized. We noticed these small music venues sprouting up over the city and we felt excited to have something that we and our kids could do together. Tim, who was twelve years old, had a guitar band, and the other kids were old enough to help make candles for the tables to assist in popping corn, to fill the glasses with juices, and they even baked a cake every week. Twice a week we and others entertained for the Northwestern College community and other Fellowship members.

But the dark night of winter 1971 brought that to an end. When some of the college students as well as Fellowship members questioned our use of too many secular songs, we bristled.

Eunice and I felt that music had to portray all the "stuff" of life, the good and the bad; secular and sacred have to be wed in order for life to blend. With the emergence of the charismatic movement within the Fellowship, Eunice and I felt perhaps the time had come for us to pull out of the commune and reassess the direction of our lives.

The charismatic movement needs further amplification. I have no idea where it began, but at Reba Place we were initially influenced by a religious swell within the Catholic churches. People felt the impowering of the Spirit to speak with the authority of God. We wanted to know of such new power. A clergy from the Episcopal church volunteered to lead a small group of us in demonstrating this phenomenon. Ten or twelve of us gathered in a camp setting to learn. This is where Eunice's simple honesty confounded the wise. As we were sitting waiting for the Spirit, our teacher asked for anyone to volunteer for receiving the gift of speaking in tongues. One of the women members shyly raised her hand. "Just open your mouth and say 'Ah,'" she was told. Eunice could bear the nervous embarrassment no longer and burst into laughter. At the same moment there were others who felt awkward and wanted to express themselves. Of course, Eunice was ashamed initially, but it allowed a good discussion of what we were doing and expecting, and we all felt good that it happened just that way.

Reba Place felt it needed to understand better the whole area of mental health. Our association with a psychiatrist at the University of Illinois by the name of Dr. Mowrer provided us with a challenge that we were not quite prepared for. Dr. Mowrer asked whether we could provide care and housing, a kind of "half-way house," to Katherine. So she moved into the rooms available in the rear of the second floor of our house at 714 Reba Place. After several months we and the Zooks, who lived in the front three rooms of the second floor, learned to know Katherine quite well. On one particular day when I was visiting with Ann upstairs, the two of us had an uneasy feeling about Katherine. As I was leaving to go to the first floor I told Ann, "Why don't you have the doctor's phone number handy, just in case."

It wasn't two hours later that I heard a very strange thumping on the floor above, as though someone were kicking on the floor. I ran up to Ann, and we decided to knock on Katherine's door to see if she needed help. Indeed she did. She was slumped over the table with a kitchen knife in her bosom. As the emergency crew was carrying her out to the ambulance, the children were just returning from school, so there was a ready audience to the crisis. The doctor called a little later and reported that Katherine had died.

The decision to leave the Fellowship was not easy. The sharing of our finances using the welfare standard allowed for few excesses, but all bills including medical were covered by the church. We didn't mind the frugal style of living. Our bonding with the members was real which made our separation more painful. In spite of a rather tight budget, the Fellowship offered us money and a car. We accepted the '67 Ford and then began the challenge of where to move. We wanted to locate somewhere within rail commuting for Don's teaching position in Evanston. Bill and Alice Howenstine whom we knew invited us to come to McHenry, fifty miles north. Val and Joe Gitlin from Woodstock had visited with a sister at the Fellowship and thus we had become acquainted with them and that area north.

The clincher was an ad that Don placed in the Geneva, Woodstock, McHenry newspapers. A spinster lady, Mrs. Wright, answered our ad and we agreed to rent her twenty-two-acre farm on the edge of Woodstock, at the convergence of Burbank and East Streets, for $250.00 a month. But at age forty, we were starting over with just a one-month's check and a used car to our name, no savings or credit, but a lot of verve and nerve and six kids.

Our immediate thought was to spend this time "in the desert" in meditation and thoughtful consideration of possibly returning again to Evanston and the commune. With Eunice's creative genius we survived on having a summer children's camp, Eunice's guitar lessons and breadmaking, and my monthly salary. We acquired a barn full of animals by carefully scanning the ads—horses, chickens, ducks, rabbits, sheep, goats—and before we knew it we were farming again...for fun!

Don was still teaching school in Evanston, a fifty-mile drive rather than a three-hour train ride. I began teaching guitar at home through the college and we were enjoying life as we gradually found friends. Then another jolt! After two years at 536 Burbank, our landlord said she needed to double our rent because I was earning money in the house by teaching guitar. I got this phone call during one of my lessons with two dear children, the Boppart girls. I burst into tears, then controlled myself. When the parents came to pick up the children, Joan, a local real estate broker, sensed something was wrong. She had no idea we did not own the property and her wheels began to spin. To make a long story short, we bought a property she had listed at 528 East Calhoun, and moved in November 1975.

It took some explaining for us to convince the Bopparts that a man of forty in the teaching profession would not have any assets and thus no down payment. No problem. Joan and Gene drew up a contract that fit our budget and the rest is history. Again Eunice's genius propelled us, as much by her soul as by her talent. She had private students who paid her

$20.00 per hour for a guitar lesson, but in reality all they wanted on a particular day was to talk to her about a bad marriage. She could teach a college class of twenty just as easily as she could a single student.

Eunice was a home decorator with no degree in design, and no money to buy new or expensive materials. She was known far and wide as the woman who made an art out of garage-sale buying. Sophisticated friends would marvel at how she could arrange a house full of junk to make it attractive enough to be on the front page in the Chicago Tribune. She was a major chef with no recipes. How people craved her homemade bread. She made the complicated, simple. She could come with a delicacy in a moment with the bare necessities. The commune living gave her some practice at developing tasty foods with little money, even for groups of twenty or more. Her passion was to invite a half dozen friends for a dinner, set tables at four or five different locations in the house for the various courses, then end with a flurry at the fireplace for a cherry jubilee. Sometimes the jubilee didn't work, but there was always a substitute in the wings. Never would we end the evening without a game of some kind. She would always suggest a prayer of thanks before the meal.

I guess it was her charisma that inspired me and others. That's why her children's programs were so successful. She used her intuition to guide her in choosing the right activity or song for different occasions.

For example, when we entertained Pete Seeger in our home in November 1991, Eunice began the concert with Pete on our stage. She handed him a yo-yo for him to use with a song she had prepared. Apologetically, Pete said, "I'm sorry I can't manage this with my arm cast." (Pete was nursing a carpal injury.) Without batting an eye and not wasting a second, she said, "O.K. Here is a bull's nose; put it on your face and we'll sing one of your own songs." And with that she broke into "I had a rooster and the rooster pleased me...."

During that same visit, Pete enjoyed walking around the garden as Eunice was showing off her joys. As she led him to the little guest house out back, she played a little ditty for him on the toy piano. Pete admired the sound, so she gave him the 2' high by 2' wide piano after etching her name in the back. The next day when I took Pete to the airport, we hugged "Good-byes" and he sauntered up to the counter with a banjo and guitar in one hand, while in the other was his suitcase and a big plastic bag containing a piano.

**"...she was the spirit of grandmother's love.
She could hear the beat of the drum and
celebrate the gifts of the spirit.
Her drum beat moved us by
loving, giving, encouraging, nudging,
pushing, pulling, smiling, hugging,
winking, and beckoning.
When her heart beat like the
drum, there wasn't a person who could say
'No' to her passion."**
- Karen Whaples

It's time to poke him again! Yep, he said I should tape record him to prove he's snoring. I'm tired. It's 11:00.

Eunice digresses from this narrative. Her diagnosis of breast cancer came in July 1991. Together we appeared at the Woodstock Memorial Hospital for a scheduled biopsy. For five years or more she had been scheduling regular recommended mammograms and been receiving a clean bill of health each time. Occasionally, over the past two years she had become suspicious of a growing lump in her left breast, but with each doctor exam she was assured there was no sign of a tumor. The doctor's report in brief states:

> "This 57-year-old female was recently evaluated in my office at the request of Dr. Lesser for an abnormality of the left breast. The patient states she has had a strange sensation in the breast for quite some time. Approximately 7-8 months ago, she developed occasional erythematous changes in the left breast. At that time reportedly, there was no palpable abnormality and a mammogram was obtained which revealed no evidence of malignancy. Subsequent to that time, however, she has continued to have erythematous changes from time to time in the left breast, and now has a palpable mass in the superior aspect of the left breast...."

So on this July 8, 1991 Eunice was insisting on a biopsy. She signed the initial papers permitting surgery if that appeared necessary to Dr. Lynd. She had great confidence in her surgeon who was well respected by our nurse friends. When Dr. Lynd and Dr. Lesser approached me in the waiting room with the news that Eunice had received a mastectomy, I was in a state of shock. I slumped over her hospital bed and sobbed with her.

Her suspicions were confirmed. Of course, we were to wait for the results of the tests, but I now trusted Eunice's intuitions implicitly. The doctor's report continued:

> "The residual tumor in its largest extent measures 2 cm. Final diagnosis: Left breast carcinoma. Left breast biopsy followed by left breast mastectomy, radical with axillary node dissection. This is a 57-year-old female who was admitted for a breast biopsy. This was positive. She underwent immediate mastectomy and axillary node dissection. Final diagnosis was that of diffusely infiltrating poorly-differentiated ductal and, in part, lobular carcinoma, left breast with metastatic tumor present in 17 out of 28 lymph nodes. The patient tolerated the procedure well. Recovery

was uneventful. Metastatic evaluation revealed no other abnormalities. She was discharged to be followed up by chemotherapy and radiation therapy...."

The cold reality gripped us like a winter night. The days and weeks that followed were a jumble of fast moving events. CANCER...REALLY...ME? We read all the available booklets, saw all the recommended tapes, heard all the daily dribble of news about "Make sure you get a regular mammogram....If you can just detect it early enough...." Rubbish! Oh, how we aired our anger and frustration, cried our pent-up tears, and prayed for deliverance. Eunice, of course, was a model patient. Mixing laughter and tears she showed me how to live, while dying. We had, and still do, a community of friends here in Woodstock who continued loving and supporting throughout the whole ordeal. I wanted the best medical advice money could buy.

Our oncologist nurse in Woodstock arranged for us to get second and third opinions from the University of Madison Medical School and also from the hospital at the University of Milwaukee. Not satisfied, I called Mayo Clinic for an observation appointment. We knew our insurance would not pay the bill for this excursion, but it didn't matter. The results of these three hospital visits concurred that the best scientific treatment for breast cancer is chemotherapy and radiation. The telephone conversations with the doctor at Dayton's Kettering hospital in Ohio confirmed our belief that other advanced therapies were not advisable for a person of Eunice's age.

Later, during a winter visit to see our children in California, we arranged to meet with the oncologist at the Scripps Hospital in San Diego to be assured there was no new discovery that would be available to us. The verdict was the same.

A lot has happened since I last wrote in this book. What an unbelievable experience to try to live a normal life while knowing my prognosis for recovery is not good. To say, "Each day is more precious" is not really true for me because I always treasured each day and new experience. When I see depressed people I feel so sorry for them; it must be worse than cancer. That's one reason I hate to complain about my predicament. I've had so many rich experiences in my sixty years. I feel so inadequate to express myself, even though my main fault is that I often talk too much.

July 1993: We're in the plane overlooking the Rockies. It's unbelievable that we're on our way to Alaska because of the generosity of our children. Thank you, kids. We've been on a month-long roller coaster ride, one rich experience after another. We've been so blessed with friends; it seems like we're eating at someone's home every night. Co, our daughter Colleen, and her fiancé Tom came to spend time with us again this summer between their assignments on the ship. She is working up to the position of chief cook or steward and loves her job. Tom painted the whole house and Colleen just pampered me and we shared hours of good talk, cards and more cards, work and more work, food and more food, and some struggles as we watched them struggle with their alcohol problem.

Then Peter and Tim came home for a visit. What a surprise! Tim hadn't been home for eight years. It was fun to see him look around the house and more fun to "jam" with him again. That was a highlight when we all sang and played guitar together. The year that Tim, Peter, and Hans traveled with me to Evanston for guitar lessons was rich beyond dreams and I'm so proud of their efforts during that time. So playing with them during this summer in the home we created for music was a memory I'll carry with me to my grave. That's only too real for me now as I contemplate the end of life. I really hate to go, but I try to stay as positive as my spirit allows.

> "The bustle in a house the morning after death
> Is solemnest of occasion enacted upon earth;
> The sweeping up the heart and putting love away
> We shall not want to use again until eternity."
> - *Emily Dickinson*

When Peter comes home, all of his old friends from town "smell" his presence and they descend on the place like bees to honey. It was so neat to hear Tim and Pete duo on the guitars. Then when we were sitting down to dinner the first night, Tim strolled in with Dean and his two kids, Jake and Kayleigh. What a surprise! Jill was the only one of the kids not present, but she had been here with her family the year before. (Now she's divorcing Jeff because of his alcohol problem.)

I had to hang loose during the summer when my dear children didn't act as I wanted them to. I reminded myself that they're not puppets, and I don't want them to be. For the most part I'm very proud of them, but the only curse we have is the alcohol party syndrome. If only they'd realize that significant fun can occur without alcohol. I suppose they got the partying spirit from us.

We've been tickled to death that Peter has made an important decision to give up the booze and he says he has never been happier in his life. He gives credit to the California laws pertaining to DUI. The penalty of money and jail was enough to show the folly of it, and he quit... cold turkey!

Don and I were so indoctrinated to fear alcohol by our Mennonite upbringing that we shun overindulgence zealously. I say overindulgence because Don and I enjoy a good glass of wine with dinner. What fun to have had six children and to now sit back and watch them grow. What fun, I say now. Don't you forget it, kids; it wasn't a party. I think I was near death several times, especially the firstborn, Dean. But I'm so glad for that boy now. I know, as a parent, alcohol has ruined relationships both between the children and us, and between our children and their spouses. It is a monster that needs to be conquered by each individual.

You kids have been so kind to call and write frequently. I remember the Mother's Day note Peter sent to me:

"A long time ago I was sitting outside on a rock
when an elf came up to me and said,
'Give me your mother, and I'll give you a pony.'
Now I was tempted, Mom, because
I had always wanted a pony,
but then I thought of how lonely
the house would be without you, so I said,
'No.'

Then he said, 'Give me your mother,
and I'll give you a brand-new bicycle
with long streamers and a loud horn.'
Boy, that sounded nice,
but then I thought of how you
were there to tuck me in at night, so I said,
'No.'

Finally he turned red in the face and said, 'Well, what in the whole world would you trade your mom for?' And I thought real hard and then told the truth. 'I wouldn't trade her for anything,' and you know what? That's still true today. I love you, Mom....
Your son, Peter"

So the summer of 1993 was interrupted by this unexpected trip to Alaska, thanks to our kids. And we found ourselves in Vancouver. It was Dean's suggestion that we stay at the Blue Horizon Hotel and what a lovely choice. The twenty-fifth floor would not have been my choice, but we had a lovely two-sided view of the city, the water, and the sky from our balcony. We had arranged to meet Tom and Colleen at the hotel.

Any minute we were expecting Colleen and Tom to come to the room, so Don had prepared the video camera to start running when he heard the knock. They arrived. We shouted, "Come in," as the camera started rolling. In walked Tom followed by Colleen who was noticeably drunk.

As we learned later, when Colleen saw the camera, that clinched her desire to never drink again and at this writing three years later, Colleen is still "on the wagon," going regularly to AA meetings and developing a new way of living through the principles of the AA program.

We were so sorry for them and for us; cause I love Colleen so much, and I know how much she hurt. All we could do was give her our love and strength.

> "Love is eternal...and love is immortal,
> and death is only a horizon,
> and a horizon is nothing
> save the limits of our sight.
> There is a land of the living
> and a land of the dead
> and the bridge is love,
> the only survival,
> the only meaning."
> - *Wilder*

The night seemed long, and with the morning came the rain. Again we waited for them for breakfast, but Colleen soon called and said she would meet us after breakfast; she needed to collect herself. Don and I found a quiet corner in the restaurant, sipped coffee, and talked very candidly about my approaching death. How shall we divide the furniture and all our treasures? We try to live positively but know we must be practical. At least that's the way I have to deal with it.

We have read so many books that try to tell us how to handle the scare of cancer. We feel so grateful that none of our kids seems greedy about our stuff. I thank God for that, because I've heard so often how families were torn apart by the distribution of an estate. We resolved that Colleen had to heal her body before we could plan very much with them. Before long Colleen arrived and amid hugs and kisses, we all healed again.

Colleen took the first step in admitting that she needed help. Over the years Eunice and I have wondered whether we needed to exercise more "tough love" for situations like this. The rain stopped and we saw the sun again. How appropriately!

> "You can give without loving,
> but you cannot love without giving."
> - *Amy Carmichael*

What a wonderful day. All are well again. Tom left for his home in Seattle and we were glad to be alone with Colleen to talk, laugh, cry if we wanted. We did all of that as we jumped a cruise bus and saw the city. At the end of the day and another nice restaurant we walked home and I nursed my poor aching knees. I guess it's just arthritis, although every pain reminds me of cancer. I made the decision that for these two weeks I would not take any chemo; Doctor Ritzman said it's up to me. I am ecstatic about the beauty of this world, and for our kids who paid for this luxurious trip.

Well, I guess I must write this page. I don't want to but I promised myself I wouldn't hide the "warts." Otherwise, it sounds too much like the class letters we continue to receive from our high school and college friends who now have grown children who are either missionaries, doctors, or college professors. Don has threatened to write one about our family, spilling all the guts. Is our society so accustomed to "whited sepulchers" that people are insecure to tell the truth? What causes us to hide our "warts" and to pretend a lie? To not write the truth feels like I'm enabling bad behavior. Anyway, last night we waited and waited for Tom to come back from Seattle where he was getting his new teeth. Finally, we left a message at our hotel and went to a nearby restaurant to eat. We tried to be positive, but Colleen was beginning to believe that Tom was on a drinking binge like she had been the night before.

Colleen was devastated that our trip, cancer and all, was initiated by these events. We decided to sleep on it, and make a decision the next day. The morning brought us all to the conclusion that we will not be controlled by Tom's behavior, so we explored the city some more. By evening we returned to the hotel and discovered Tom had returned...drunk. What now? He was sorry, of course, but we remembered Gamble Rogers telling us at a storyteller's camp, "Sorry is as sorry does." The dark of night arrived and with it the hope that the morning would bring new promises.

"Nothing can make up for the absence of
someone whom we love.
It is nonsense to say that God fills the gap;
He doesn't fill it, but on the contrary,
He keeps it empty and so helps us to keep alive
our former communion with each other,
even at the cost of pain.
The dearer and richer our memories,
the more difficult the separation.
But gratitude changes the pangs of memory
into a tranquil joy.
The beauties of the past are borne,
not as a thorn in the flesh,
but as a precious gift themselves."
- *Dietrich Bonhoeffer*

The morning brought us together again with Colleen visibly shaken. After a long talk with Tom they resolved to stay together and work it out. They will seek counseling and do whatever it takes to stay away from alcohol. Tom will report to us at breakfast....What do we think, Colleen wondered. I asked her to open herself to God's light. She said she already feels God's strength, but needs others too. I've always been thankful for:

> "One day at a time, dear Jesus.
> That's all I'm askin' from you....
> Just give me the strength to do every day
> What I have to do....
> Yesterday's gone, dear Jesus,
> And tomorrow may never be mine....
> So for today, show me the way,
> One day at a time."

I feel my body getting weaker from the buildup of fluid in my lungs. I can hardly walk without feeling like I'm dragging a weight. My breathing is shallow; I can't sneeze or cough without sharp pain. I'm trying to let go and have a wholesome feeling about dying. I have a real curiosity about experiencing the other side. Don and I cry together and have shared to the depths. I'm relieved to know that I can sleep well through it all...no chemo, just cancer! That means a lot, and I still love to eat and play cards. Co came over late last night after nursing Tom and we played and laughed. We needed the outlet bad.

Next morning. We're up and raring to go. Don's had his early morning walk with paper and coffee. I stayed and watched "Good Morning" show. We're all ready to "face the music" with Tom's speech and his new teeth that we haven't seen yet. The weather looks great out there and we're packed ready to board the ship for Alaska... can't wait. Co just called and Tom isn't ready to see us, so the three of us will go by ourselves to Gastown section of Vancouver, look around and have breakfast. We'll drive the rented jeep so we have transportation back to the hotel to get our bags at departure time. We shopped, talked, and laughed for a couple hours.

Soon it was time for Co and Don to return to get Tom and our bags at the hotel. I found a stationery store where I looked for an appropriate card to give Co and Tom when we board the ship.

Within a half hour, sure enough, they had returned with Tom, new teeth and all, but no word about his forays. I was uncomfortable till Co finally asked Tom to tell us how he's feeling about everything. Of course, he's very sorry and has decided to take a certain pill that would make him violently ill if he drank. In addition he wants to begin going to AA with Co. Nice talk! They love each other so much. "When will they ever learn; when will they ever learn?"

We parted for the ship in each other's arms, crying and wishing them God's blessing. Co seems so genuinely appreciative of us and the example we gave to them. This is the first week of her new life in AA.

"Hope is the thing with feathers
that perches on the soul,
that sings the song without the words,
and never stops at all."
- *Emily Dickinson*

As Eunice and I were told, when alcoholics kick the habit their life begins as though it is their first year. The bonding of Eunice and Colleen was an enormous mountain climbed. From the summer of 1991 when cancer was first discovered their relationship blossomed, but the Vancouver experience, as painful as it was for all of us, was the Higher Power kicking in, and solid resolutions formed.

Bon Voyage Alaska.

We found our cabin much more spacious than I expected, with two portholes. Time to go for food, which was a-plenty! The buffet was great! We ate on the deck and watched the towns glide by, even had a nap and just watched people. Then we walked slowly around the whole ship and lounged until dinner. The dark and the quiet of night came quickly. At 4:00 a.m., I got awake. My mind was racing uncomfortably so I prayed and collected myself. I brought a book for just these times: *The Girl* by Meribel La Frier.

Morning arrived...still no icebergs. But there was a good breakfast. Among the 900 passengers we suddenly spied a lady with a familiar-looking shirt. The lettering read "Holly-Woodstock." The Langs from our town, Woodstock, Illinois. So we haven't escaped quite. More lounging on the deck and talking about the events in Vancouver and our upcoming estate sale. What shall we do with the Singalong in September which is publicized as a celebration of my life? I don't know how I'm going to deal with it. We plan to move out of our house into the garage which we will convert into living space.

Cancer almost seems like a diversion. We heard a short lecture on Alaska and its history. The scenery is beautiful, but after while I started getting oceanbound. I love walking, but my bum knee is painful. I try to keep my spirits up and not whine too much. Don is so good to me. Occasionally I feel a panic with the thought of "What would I do if I can't breathe....There's no hospital....I know the fluid is building up in my lungs again." Don and I checked out the emergency treatment centers on board which at least are adequate.

I'm thoroughly enjoying just being me with no responsibilities. It's very strange here so far from home; so much time to think about the life Don and I have had with our children, friends, and music; the years on the farm, the publishing house, college; life in the commune in Evanston; the year in Campus, Illinois, where we were treated like a minority for befriending blacks; the Hootenanny in Evanston; the hard decision to move out of the commune to Woodstock; the years without a savings or assets except our love for each other (That's an asset I don't take for granted when I hear all the bickering going on between married couples); the Woodstock friends that have continued to support us; the three trips to Russia; and visiting our kids in California and Hawaii. I think of cancer constantly, and of our darling kids whom I'll miss when I cross Jordan; each of them is so special. I wish I could tell them how to avoid the pitfalls.

It's hard to break into this reverie, and I don't do it with dry eyes. Eunice has been a phenomenal mother and wife and friend. The events she enumerates could not have been done without considerable venturesome spirit, maybe even reckless abandon. Our connections with the American Friends Service Committee and the Experiment in International Living afforded us some of these experiences without cost to us.

One such experience was the summer of 1967 when we led a group of high school kids with AFSC to Philo, California. These two months we were part of the staff of Clear Water Ranch, a home for disturbed children. Eunice with her guitar was especially influential in reaching the children. One particular autistic boy would always lounge on the deck of the main building. After many days of constantly playing her guitar near where Jimmy was crouched, Eunice saw him gradually become more and more interested in the guitar music. On one occasion he began trying to say something, but we could never see further progress because our stay had ended. I've often wondered what little miracles she accomplished in her life through sharing with others her enthusiasm for music. In most situations, Eunice tried to make a difference.

"When we do the best we can,
we never know what miracle is wrought in our life,
or in the life of another."
- Helen Keller

She talks to our children....

I guess the pitfalls are for a reason. It's so exciting to watch you mature, make mistakes and pick up the pieces and move ahead. Jill, I get overwhelmed when I think of you going to school and raising three kids while holding a job. Peter, we're so proud of how you turned your life around. Tim, you have such a wonderful gift of music. Tears are in my eyes as I write this. What a neat experience to sing and play with you this summer in our home, and thanks for sharing so deeply. You have a neat family. Dean, because of your generosity and "need," we were lucky to get to know you and Jake and Kayleigh so much better. What wonderful memories of the winters at your house. Co, you don't deserve to have had to go through such tough times. You're too good of a person, but now I believe you're on a new path. You have so much to offer people. Hans babe, why do I love to tease you so much?

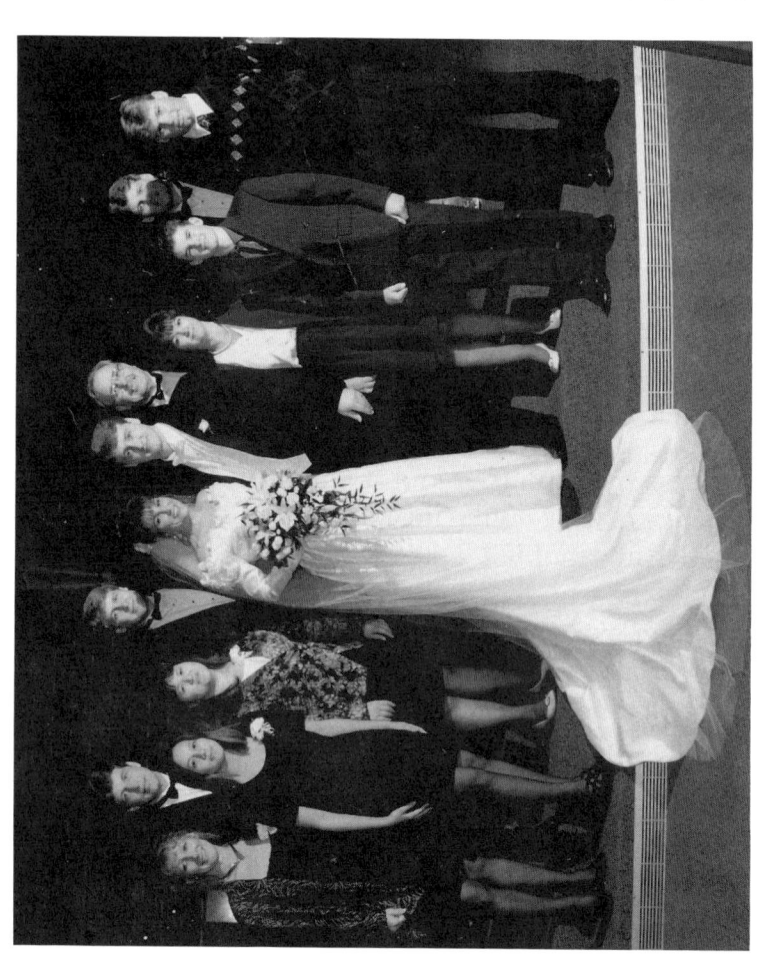

Left to right: Colleen, Dean, Stephanie (Jill's daughter), Jill, Peter, Sherry, Hans, Don, Holly (Tim's wife), Bryan (Tim's son), Tim, and Jason (Holly's son). Credit: M.E. Studios.

Cause you're my baby and always will be. What a neat kid! We're proud of you, going through those years in school, and those decisions about who to marry. That's what's fun about having so many kids. Each one is so different and special in so many ways. Hans, I've been so happy that you have been so friendly to my many friends who stop in, more than you wish they would, I'm sure. And, of course, your friend Sherry, we love her too. I'm getting tired, diary....

A note from Colleen:

"Mom, you were my mother, but you became my friend. You taught me to be strong, to embrace life, and that love is important. Your appreciation and love of Dad, friendship, music, candlelight, chocolates, bargains, beautiful days, and life itself has been inspiring. You left this earth and all you love with the same acceptance and trust in God and love for adventure that you lived by. I won't miss you too much since you've taken up permanent residence in my heart. I love you."

- Colleen

And a note from Dean:

"What a rich experience to have "Pa Pa" and Grandma, with her bag of "tricks," living with Kayleigh, Jake, and me. Each year we looked forward to their visit during the winter months. The smell of fresh baked bread cooling off in the kitchen and candles glowing in every nook and cranny. Each Christmas was festive with bubbles and music in the air. Grandma and the children spent countless hours by the fire singing and acting out songs with puppets every evening. I really got to know and appreciate Mom during those 'Fallbrook years.' She had the secret to happiness and shared it with all she met. She still lives with us...."   - Dean

"I am of the opinion that my life belongs to the community, and as long as I live, it is my privilege to do for it whatever I can. I want to be thoroughly used up when I die, for the harder I work, the more I live. Life is no brief candle to me, it is a sort of splendid torch which I have got hold of for a moment, and I want to make it burn as brightly as possible before handing it on to future generations."   - *George Bernard Shaw*

Well, I didn't write for awhile because we're having too much fun. Brief stop at Skagway. Came back to the cabin, took a nap and had "high tea" out on the deck, then a lecture on Sitka, the next town. Played a hand of bingo and made the mistake of sitting in the front row where a director saw me and wanted to dance. If he only knew. At last, snow-capped mountains of beauty. The little towns where we stop for day tours are exquisite. I couldn't resist buying an eagle puppet. I have a fascination with eagles. The eagles are endangered because of the build-up of pesticides in their bodies from the contaminated fish. What does that say about us humans? We came home worn-out and went to sleep in each other's arms. Saw musicians in Juneau and heard about the Russian ancestors.

Night arrived before I wanted it to. It's those hours of dark that cause me to worry about my shortness of breath; will I find a hospital? I don't like to repeat these anxieties to Don all the time; he's been so patient and understanding; it's getting worse each day.

The next day came and I'm still here. Juneau is a cute little town built up by the gold rush. I love the histories of these places. Oh yes, I forgot to tell you of Dolly's Museum in Ketchikan, the most famous brothel along the pass. They charged $3.00 a "trick" and Dolly didn't quit for the day until she had earned $75.00—a hefty sum in those days. In Juneau it rained, so one of the tours was canceled; however, we did take a bus to the glacier. That was exciting. Also, we stopped to watch the salmon spawning, then dying. Dinners on board are too elegant and fun. You order anything and as much as you want from the menu. The waiter and busboy are hilarious, one French and the other Turkish. There are maybe 500 people at one sitting. Don insists I should buy something for myself at the next town. I'll stop now and read a very interesting book I bought about the Klondike Gold Rush.

One day moves into the next so fast that sometimes two days have passed since I last wrote. Ship docked at 6:00 a.m. in Sitka, a small fishing village; almost reminds me of a small Austrian village Don and I visited in 1973 when we made a whirlwind tour of Europe. Small boats (tenders) shuttle us to land where we are on our own as to how much we want to tour. First we took a bus tour of the town, stopping at a dance hall where we were entertained by a youth dancing group...Russian-style dress and music, because of earlier Russian settlements. It reminded me of our visits to Russia in 1984, 1988, and 1990.

Eunice and I first traveled to Russia in 1984 without the luxury of a tour. There were some frightening moments. For instance, on one occasion as we were riding the train from Moscow to Warsaw, the train came to a gradual stop in some desolate area and we saw several border patrols entering the train. Before long there was a knock on our bunk door and a swarthy-looking English-speaking officer asked us for passports and visas, then began rummaging through our bags. He was baffled by the Pennsylvania Dutch souvenir we had packed as a gift, and we were just as baffled in trying to explain what it was. He was further intrigued by our Sony tape recorder. He asked me to turn it on, and he was rewarded with a song Eunice and I were singing: "Here's a land full of power and glory," by Phil Ochs. He smiled and asked, "This is you?" He took the tapes, and we didn't see them again.

In 1988 we traveled with a group of about 100 Americans joined by a similar number of Russians on board the "Gorky" on the Volga River for two weeks. But the most spectacular experience was the two weeks living with Sergei and Tanya Nikitin in the summer of 1990. A strange coincidence occurred on that trip. We flew into London, then had to wait a few days for our Moscow flight so we decided it'd be fun to drive to Wales. (On a trip to the U.K. in 1984 we had driven through parts of England, took a bus through Northern Ireland down to Dublin, but always wished that we had stopped longer in Wales. Now's our chance.) We didn't have a distinct location, but the main road out of London appeared to head northwest, so we followed it to the border to a quaint-looking town in northern Wales by the name of Llangollen. Intrigued by what appeared to be downtown, we stopped the first passer-by and asked if there was any music going on that night. We knew the Welsh were premier singers. Without any hesitation, the chap answered in a definite English accent, "There's the Eistedfodd." He explained that this was the week of the annual international music competition—even Pavrotti once sang here. I guess we lucked out! After dropping our bags at a convenient bed and breakfast, we drove north of town, enjoying the rolling hills.

About two miles out of town we noticed a demolished building that was shaped like an abbey, with cows grazing in the surrounding fields and neatly mowed grass at the base of the rubble. A few visitors were roaming the ruins. It looked like the ideal spot for Eunice and me to sit and practice some tunes. So we touted our guitar and autoharp to a distant part of the complex and started singing. Before long a middle-aged couple sauntered up, waited till we were done singing then introduced themselves. Should we be surprised to learn he was a professor at Columbia University in New York, a teacher of English to foreign students? When he learned that we were enroute to Russia, he spoke of having a Russian student whom he was tutoring presently. Could we believe that Zenya Kiperman, his student, was the very person whom we had spoken to on the phone about our visit to the Nikitins because Sergei had given us his number? To further blow our minds, this professor lived along the Hudson River, a neighbor of Pete Seeger. Well, the summer had only begun, and already we felt strange coincidences.

The Eistedfodd had one other more humbling experience. As we sat in the huge tent listening to the singers, we kept watching a strange-looking "quasimodo"-type person who would always appear to be watching us; it got a little scary, but then we brushed it off as perhaps just another needy person who finds solace in music. We awoke in the morning with our B&B hosts at breakfast to find that the only other person at the table with us was "quasimodo."

The two days we stayed in Llangollen were not enough, but we had to get back to London for our plane connection to Moscow. There is not nearly enough space to tell the Russian story completely, but I'll share some tidbits.

Sergei and Tanya Nikitin met us at the airport and drove us to their apartment near Moscow University. We met Sergei's mother, Mira, who lives with them, and their eighteen-year-old son Sasha. The three-room apartment was small, but we all managed to have some privacy for those two weeks. Mira ruled supreme in the 6'x6' kitchen, but Eunice begged to prepare one of the meals for which she had stowed some canned Chicago ham and picked up other necessary vegetables and breads at the Moscow market. This special meal, of course, would be a party in true Eunie style even to the end-of-meal game.

Tanya's parents, members of the Communist Party, were also present as we sat down to a beautifully decorated table with candles, of course, and Russian vodka. The meal was delicious and the "Pin the tail on the donkey" was won by (who else) Sergei.

Other trip highlights were the side trips to special dachas and little villages. Eunice's creative talents and love with the Russian people was absorbing. We attended the annual folk festival along the Volga River with our Nikitin friends, who are part of a committee to secure talent for the festival attended by 50 to 75,000 people from all over Russia. There were several stages and Eunice was the entertainer at one of the stages with several thousand people sitting on the ground. She called for six children volunteers from the crowd and won a wondrous applause as she led them through the "Rooster" song. The final event of the weekend was the night concert where Eunice and I were invited along with a dozen other finalists. The stage was in the shape of a guitar floating on the inlet while the audience sat on the mountainside. Eunice also appeared on Russian television with a group of children who were delighted by her warmth and love.

We're still in Alaska. There are still many reminders of Russia's past here in Sitka. Next we visited the eagle and owl sanctuary, a hospital that cares for injured birds. One eagle in particular had been in captivity so long it began to "imprint"...that is, it attaches itself to a human by following that person around, trying to mate because the eagle thinks the human is its mother.

The American eagle was always a fascination for Eunice. So it is not surprising that the visit to the bird sanctuary was an important stop. Not long after we returned home from the trip, Eunice was alone in the music room practicing her guitar as was her custom. She would love to go from one instrument to another when she had the room all to herself so she wouldn't bother anyone. On this particular day as she was creating music she was astonished to observe an eagle landing on our deck railing not fifteen feet away...an eagle, mind you. Eunice was transfixed! Never did we see in Woodstock an eagle making a pit stop of this kind. She didn't want to stop playing in case the eagle would fly away. She wanted to watch it forever. Within five minutes it spread its huge beautiful wings and flew away. Eunice slumped into a chair nearby and turned on the TV to get a diversion from her ecstasy, thinking perhaps she was dreaming. She flipped the dial to a talk show. The host of the show was introducing a naturalist who was demonstrating (are you ready for this?) the beauty and the habits of the American eagle. With this view of an eagle right before her on the screen, she made the unmistakable comparison with the one that had just appeared before her on the deck. Eunice sat me down when I returned home and shocked me with her story of the eagle's visit. Was it a sign, she asked? She hid the thought within her that the eagle was the messenger telling her of her own impending flight, for six months later she died of cancer.

I did some quick shopping and then back to the ship where we enjoyed a scrumptious meal and watched whales spouting. The last night on ship was billed as a "formal." Don and I usually don't fit in those settings. In certain moods, I would have gone anyway, even with my "garage sale" wardrobe, but we've been filled to the gills and ready to vegetate. We read and talked and wrote letters, or I should say, I wrote the letters because Don was sick. As the ship left the Inside Passage and sailed towards Anchorage over open sea, it got very rough. The pills helped Don through the high seas and morning arrived by the time I had fallen asleep.

Don brought me breakfast in bed that last morning before disembarking. What more can I say about the trip. It was unforgettable. And now I'm ready to face the next chapter in my short life, home and chemotherapy and nausea and fear. I know it's bitter/sweet because I'm sure I won't live through another summer, but I've learned a simple lesson from my granddaughter, Kayleigh. When I left her in California the spring of 1993, I was tucking her in bed and said, "Kayleigh, Grandma is leaving in the morning and I won't see you again for a long time, why aren't you crying?" She shrugged and said, "That's life." And so it is for all of us....Life then death...then the mystery!

I've not said much about my wonderful husband. Except for a few warts, I could not have found a better man anywhere in the universe! Where I was weak, he was strong. Starting from the first days of our marriage, we needed to sift out the excessive baggage from our ancestors; doesn't everyone need to do that? I would usually be gullible and believe it all, whereas Don would help evaluate the contents. However, when it came to being sensitive, I was his guru. He didn't like confrontations of sad, crying discussions. His tendency was to hide them under a rug and pray that things would get better later. However, we had one good thing in our favor. We always wanted to choose the right way together, sometimes on our knees. We didn't ever want to go to bed mad at each other. He learned to let me cry, and to let me get it out. I could pout quite well, and it finally worked for both of us.

I had such a serious problem at the beginning of our marriage because Don enjoyed playing ball too much, I thought. Our church at home frowned on playing ball too competitively. Don was used to lots of sports. And worst of all, the men wore "shorts" to play basketball, and we women would sit there and watch. I was brought up to understand where the sin borderline was. That really made life very simple.

In Mennonite circles in our youth there were differences in taboos, depending on what part of the country you lived. Eastern Mennonites were more conservative than those living west of Ohio. Then there were pockets of Mennonites in the Lancaster, Pennsylvania, area, that were more conservative than others in the Souderton area. These differences largely had to do with the wardrobes, but there were other more subtle differences as well. This made dating across Mennonite boundaries less frequent in the early 1950's. Certainly, rarely did you see anyone dating outside the Mennonite Church. Eunice and I found ourselves in that unusual category of dating between differing Mennonite conferences...but love prevailed.

As we learned during the years 1952-1958 on our moves from eastern to western Pennsylvania to Virginia to Indiana to Illinois, we had to constantly reevaluate the bottom line. I was even embarrassed to come downstairs in a long housecoat, or wear my hair down. That looked too sexy according to my father, who would communicate his concern through my mother. Don got me through this with great patience. I was more protected from the world than Don was in the early years; although both of us attended public grade schools where differences in modes of dress and behaviors were most cutting. For example, our Mennonite upbringing instructed us to remain seated during the pledge of allegiance to the flag because of its implication in subverting the message of Jesus, "My kingdom is not of this world; if it were then would my servants fight."

Music was always a big part of our lives during our dating years in the early 1950's. Don was usually the song leader in church and often we were in quartets. Don was the director of a choir of twenty young people from the Lancaster community who traveled around to some churches.

Don's colorblindness was the butt of much teasing. In high school one day one of my friends noticed he had two different-colored socks on. They never let me forget it to this day. I still need to train him about his taste with clothes. He has enough humility to change his outfit when I ask him to. It may be wearing thin.

He and I work well together. When fixing our house we designed it together, matching each other's ideas and creating a music paradise with the recycled items nobody else wanted.

Oh yes. The trip to Alaska did come to an end with a harrowing experience. We had a nice day on ship, met some friends we had seen throughout the trip but hadn't talked to. He was a doctor whose sister-in-law had a double mastectomy. As part of the entertainment, Don and I sang "The Guest" during a talent show. We went to our final dinner and then sat on the deck and watched the glaciers, whales, and mountains as we passed Prince William Sound. Then to bed at 10:30.

Don soon fell asleep and I got into my book on the gold rush. I got to the place where they were having all the trouble with icebergs, shipwrecks, etc., until I finally fell asleep. It seemed only a few hours before I was awakened by grinding of metal, people shouting, and engines sputtering. Of course my mind was still in the book, but I was bodily awake and woke Don immediately. We couldn't see anything out of the portholes. After much fretting, Don went up a flight of stairs and discovered we had arrived at our final stop where we would board a train for

Anchorage. It was still very early, though, and we went back to sleep until "wake up" call....What a relief!

Don is reading the book Tim left with us, *Life After Life*, and he interrupts me with interesting passages. I shy away from the book and prefer to read *Klondike Fever*. Why? I believe because I can forget my serious condition. I have been reminded a lot on this trip how I'm slowly deteriorating just in these past two weeks, shortness of breath and the redness on my chest has spread a lot.

Eunice skipped over the next several days. When we left the ship we spent the day in Anchorage, boarded a plane for Seattle, changed flights for Chicago. We didn't dispute the fact that cancer spread more quickly without Eunice's reliance on chemo. It was her decision and I supported her.

August 1993: We're home. How sweet it was to see Hans at the airport at 5:00 a.m. We had a wonderful dinner at Hackman's the first night home. Also Letty, our neighbor, had flowers waiting for us, the house was clean, lots of nice mail, and a call from our son, Dean. Is this being loved or what?

We got into the rush right away. Mom and Pop called thanking us for the fish we sent them from Alaska. Lois and Martyne (my sisters) called, finished the laundry, went to Aldi to get groceries for the busy weekend coming up with the Singalong. Wetzels are coming, Mildred and Marv Landis and Bill and Marina will also be visiting....and do I have cancer? I'm trying to forget it. I'll start cooking tomorrow and freezing it because on Monday I start on chemo again and possibly won't feel good for awhile. Or shall I just enjoy the quality of life I have? The decision is mine. Don will do whatever I want and that's the way I want it to be.

Caremark was the provider of nursing care at home upon consultation with our oncologist, Dr. Ritzman. The formula for chemo treatment was assigned by our doctor, but if we chose to have a less powerful formula we could. The obvious side effects with a stronger dosage would have been much more severe. Eunice chose a 75% dose, which allowed her milder side effects and the risk of a shorter life. Upon our return from Alaska in August till the end of November Eunice was using a regular treatment of chemo for three weeks on and one week off.

"Love and pity and wish well to every soul in the world; dwell in love, and then you dwell in God; hate nothing but the evil that stirs in your own heart." *-William Law*

Nice quiet day today, Sunday. Don fixed some furniture, made some decisions about what things we would sell. He made me a wonderful breakfast in bed and then we went back to sleep till 10:30. I did my most hateful job, answering mail. Then I made a salmon steak dinner as we watched "60 Minutes." We talk a lot about leaving our stuff, what to sell, and what to give to our kids and friends. Sometimes I cry, but it also feels so right. I'm not worried that we can't enjoy life wherever we go from here, but the responsibilities of this big house have finally gotten to me. Our monthly Singalong is this weekend. Of course, there is work to do, but I need the involvement in that activity to keep my mind whole.

The Caremark nurse came to take a sample of my blood to determine with my doctor when I can start chemo. She was sure I had fluid in my lungs, so she called Dr. Ritzman and I went straightway to the hospital for chest x-rays. During my two hours there I became really ill. My best friend Esther Hackman, R.N., walked by. I didn't want her to see me crying, but I couldn't hide my fears. She comforted me, but we were all sure it meant that the cancer had spread to the lungs because I'm so short of breath and the redness on my chest has really spread!

I would hear the results the next day. Those hours seemed like days when at last the phone rang at 9:30 a.m. Dr. Lynd, my surgeon, said that they would recommend aspirating my lungs whenever I could give them the word. Horrors! He said it might have to be done several times, but yes, cancer had spread to my lungs. Tears and more tears. Don and I were not as prepared as we thought we were for this. Sometimes I just want to be left alone, and Don understands. Next morning we went out to breakfast with the Hackmans, and I felt better again.

In addition to shortness of breath, I get these constant "hot flashes." At least thirty times a night I get awake in deep sweat. Don is so patient and promises never to divorce me for it...we still try to joke our way through. I did catch him sleeping on the big chair he got from the kids for Father's Day.

Last night, I took two sleeping pills and slept great! Yesterday was a zoo here. Marian wanted so badly to come and see me. Later I found out she hoped to have a healing for me. I just thanked God for such a great life and had more the attitude "Thy will be done." I can't feel right about praying for divine healing. My God is compassionate.

"The act of dying is also one of the acts of life."
- *Marcus Aurelius*

I don't need to tell God I have cancer, do I? Don and I pray for comfort, which is a way of focusing our spirits. I can get real peace by my own reaching for that higher power and quieting myself.

A friend told me about her son's attempted suicide the other day, an ordained minister! As we were eating, Julie Hanson came and wanted to speak to me in the other room. She informed me that a mutual friend of ours had cancer. Then Phyllis came and ate a little soup. Soon the Caremark lady, Mary, came for two or three hours, and was flabbergasted at all the activity. Paul Chandley stopped in and told how he and Kay had been invited to the MET. We had pie and coffee together and then Fred Boger came to talk.

Finally, I was alone with Nurse Mary; I love her. I trust her judgment because she's honest with me, and she lets me be myself. She was plugging me into the chemo and looked up suddenly and said, "My, you have a lot of people that love you," and then she laughed. For my critics who say I shouldn't do so much, I have to say, "When you have cancer, then you decide what you want to do; as for me I'll do what I feel my spirit is calling for."

After the treatment, I quickly made a huge batch of peanut butter cookies for the committee of twenty people who were coming to discuss the future of the Singalong. What a neat group of people. They're all so excited about continuing the monthly event. Someone mentioned, "You mean it's going to take twenty people to do what Don and you have been doing for fourteen years?"

Actually, it won't be as hard for them because they won't have to take care of the outside, or clean the apartment, etc. They want so badly to keep the same open spirit that has been a part of this place. Anyone can come and perform without regard to talent. I know the AA group has been always present because it is good entertainment without liquor being served. The upshot of the meeting was that duties would be assigned to carry on the work. We would meet again on the 25th of August (my birthday) and make final plans for the September Singalong.

Today was more of the same, nice day, lots of company and I did odds and ends of jobs and cooking for the weekend. Don fixed the outside garden so nice and planted new flowers. I just called Jill; she seems so happy. I'm pleased she can keep it all together. What a job she had, and such a good attitude.

6:00 a.m...Don proved his mettle again this morning. He opened his eyes and said, "What shall I make for breakfast?" I first declined, thinking he'll need to be getting breakfast regularly soon when the chemo starts kicking in, but he insisted so I enjoyed a wonderful tray of juice, scrambled eggs, toast, bacon, coffee, and a turtle that Letty thought I needed. What a great neighbor!

Yesterday we practiced and sang for the first time in awhile. We even taped it. That was fun, but I sure don't have the stamina anymore. It's scary! Now a new wrinkle started today. My sternum is very sore and tender...why?

I'm sitting in bed. Just finished eating and reading the paper. I'll watch the news and get up and start the day. Ha, Ha...We went back to bed and six hot flashes later got up! Don turned on some music to bake bread by, Tim and Pete singing "Free Falling." What memories of music; now to work.

The energy level Eunice continued to have after two years of cancer treatment was amazing. But this is a woman that always loved to work; there was never a maid. She loved cooking, cleaning, and the most hum-drum of housework. Yet she was the consummate entertainer and host to a party. Needless to say, she had slowed down considerably through this illness, but the drive was still there, and I knew that she wanted to use her own judgment about when to back off activities.

Days later. You'll never know, understand, or believe the human roller coaster we've been on. My sister Martyne and Conrad arrived as well as Bill and Marina. We had a great time playing games, cooking, eating. Anyone that showed up Friday had to help or watch me work, no visiting. There was raisin bread to be made for the weekend, and a huge round cake pan of canned peaches with two cans of pie apples, with a cake mix on top and baked with whipped cream. It went over big. The recipe came to me as I looked in my larder and saw what needed to be used up since we're leaving this place soon. We enjoy Marina and Bill because they fit right in with the work. Much of the conversation had to do with our immediate future. I'm glad that Don and I feel so secure in our desire to sell our household goods, rent this space out to reliable people, and live in one of our smaller units.

Well, I didn't sleep much Friday night; should have taken a sleeping pill, but I resist pills like mad. I got up early to make breakfast and felt quite good all day. We all worked together to get ready for our weekend. I am good at orchestrating the situation and ordering others around: make the punch, get the fresh flowers and put them on the two huge containers of punch, make the iced tea and juices. We sat down with Betsy Green who appeared with a rough draft design for our "Masthouse T-Shirts."

Mom just called that Pop, now eighty-eight, went to the hospital for a gall bladder operation. Amy called, suffering with a bit of manic-depression, and wanted to talk. After a leisurely breakfast between phone calls, we all got busy getting ready for the evening Singalong.

What a crowd! We must have had nearly 300 people. Here's a sampling of the music: Gerry Wayne, 87, played her usual dedicatory song about the Masthouse and then flopped with another song. She came up to me later and said a strange thing happened while playing her balalaika. Her hand wouldn't cooperate and she thinks she had a ministroke on stage. I played with an ensemble of recorders, Don and I sang some favorites, Paul and Kay played piano and sang a song dedicated to me: "Ride on Chariot." I had to cry, of course. It seems it will happen only too soon, and on and on till about 1:30 a.m. As usual a carload of us went to Crystal Lake and had hamburgers. Steve and Sylvia and Don and I needed this time together to debrief about the Singalong. We got home about 4:15 a.m., slept till 7:30, and got up to make chip beef and toast cups for the whole gang. About noon our guests left, so I slept for a few hours till the children's show.

The children started arriving for their show which went super. About fifty people showed up. I love it even though I'm wiped out by the end of the two-hour program. I have this fascination with my 100 puppets because of the joy I see those kids having.

I can't believe it's Wednesday already. I'm learning how to pace myself because of my energy level. I watch plenty of TV to relax and keep my mind from concentrating on myself. Dr. Lynd called and said he was afraid I'd hesitate to call him over the weekend, but he encouraged me to call him if I ever have any questions. Since it is so hard to reach my primary Doctor Ritzman, I'm so glad I have Dr. Lynd to rely on. Nurse Mary from Caremark came today and wanted me to talk about fears of pain or dying. She knew I was not afraid to die, but I was so scared of uncontrollable pain. She really made me feel better by explaining that I do not need to go through any pain because they can give me any dosage of morphine I want. Esther had told me the same thing. In fact Esther has been very frank with me lately; it makes me think they expect me to die or something. I truly wouldn't be surprised if I would; my redness is moving fast down my stomach. I know I have inflammatory cancer, lung cancer, and maybe bone cancer. Why shouldn't I expect to die? I want to make the most of it while I'm here, so get out of my way. I'm surprised I feel as good as I do most of the time. My breath is awfully short, and I can't always finish a sentence without taking a breath, plus it feels like I have a tight band around my chest because of the build-up of fluid. I still have a strange, grateful spirit; however, I may lose that soon if I get a lot of pain. Even if I have to die young, I feel like Don and I have had such a rich full life.

Today I made a pot of soup from a wonderful piece of beef that Martyne had brought me. Then Betsy Green showed up for lunch. She wants to do this artwork for our upcoming tape because she needs to show her love for me and she doesn't know what else to do. Letty was outside, so I invited her in to eat with us, too. The appliance man came to fix something and then Esther showed up to allay my fear about pain and then Caremark Mary came for a couple hours.

After a nap, Don and I went to Fiske's for dinner and then an evening meeting with John Howell about the Singalong committee. I began to feel tired so I went to bed and flopped. I just turned the TV on to an announcement. "A new dramatic cure for cancer." Peter called and we had a lovely talk; he is such a positive kid, so vulnerable, in a way so much like me. Marian called and said she is still praying for a cure for me. Of course, I want to be healed. "Please, God, heal me now!"

Dean called to thank us for the flowers we sent him on his fortieth birthday. He sounded so happy. Co and

Tom called three times saying how happy they are to be part of AA now and getting counseling, a dream come true; I guess it's now time for me to die. They have so much to offer others with the same problem. I can't reach Jill the last few days. Hans stopped in last night. It's fun to see him every few days. What an organization man and so excited about his law practice. I hope Hans and Sherry iron out their problems; they're a neat couple.

Some nights I don't sleep well and I suggested to Don that he get another bed, but he would have none of it. He wants to sleep with me as long as he can; there's little else to entice him these days. I try to sleep flat, then inclined, then jump up because of unbearable flashes. Finally, Don tries to find my sleeping pills that I resist, and brings me two of them. It works. I sleep for the next five hours.

This was a good day. We went to Harvard to order the T-shirts. So we made a day of it by going to find garage sales; it's still fun. Will I ever get tired of that pleasure? Then we wandered up to Wisconsin to look at RV's. We're getting so excited about buying one and now we have an idea what we want; we like the Bounder best. As much fun as I've had in this house, decorating, entertaining, it's too much for me now. I'm not nearly as worried about the future when I can consider getting rid of this big house and living in an RV. I marvel at how death doesn't worry me. Anyone who created this wonderful world and its creatures has sure got something else up "her" sleeve.

My fascination with garage sales conjures up so many memories. One joke on me occurred at our own garage sale several years ago. The day was long because I never was satisfied with a normal sale. I always prepared pancakes and other breakfast choices for our customers, to try to earn a few extra bucks. When evening approached I was just eager to get rid of things, so I began telling people just to help themselves to the tables of leftover items.

I noticed a truck in front of the house, and as I glanced out the window of our house, I saw a family looking over the yard treasures that remained. I assumed they had just arrived in the truck and was hopeful they could load all the rest of our stuff. Don had gone to help someone deliver a couch they had purchased, so I called out the door and told them to help themselves to what they wanted.

Because they appeared to be Spanish/Americans and may not have understood me, I walked out, pointed to the truck, and encouraged them to load it up with anything they wanted.

They seemed perplexed but quickly started loading tires, clothes, a couple tables, and two baskets of odds and ends. I was relieved to see Don returning just then so I went in the house and let him take over.

I arrived just in time to see Eunice going in the house and was unaware of what had transpired. As I got out of my car, Eddie, our neighbor across the street, was hustling toward me with his married son, John. He seemed a little perturbed and confused as he described how John was looking out his kitchen window and noticed these Spanish people loading things in John's truck. Eddie could see my bewilderment as well, since I did not know the truck belonged to John, nor was I aware of any problems.

At that point Eunice appeared on the porch again and quickly unraveled the events. We all had a big laugh. John assured our Spanish/American neighbors that he would deliver their goods to their house two blocks away, our front yard was cleared of garage sale left-overs, and Eddie never let me forget it. Eddie is a hard worker, often intoxicated at the end of a day, and is in awe of us, occasionally calling me Reverend.

"We say 'Good-bye' but not forevermore;
The call but summons to the further shore.
And when we too embark
It is not for the dark of unknown seas,
But for the welcome meeting with loved ones
Gone before who wait our greeting.
Living in hope and faith, we fear not death;
'Tis but the gate of life."   - *Unknown*

Eunice has always had a strong sense of Divine guidance. Not in the sense of being a puppet but of trying to live each moment in the Light, something akin to a Quaker philosophy. She and I always had a profound feeling, though, the rain falls on the just and unjust alike. Living a good spiritual life does not necessarily mean success. Although Eunice was easily bored with Bible study, special prayer meetings, church attendance and the like....she was the perfect example of living each moment in God's love and care. Fortunately, we agreed on this primary principle of the marriage of secular and sacred into a united front. Every moment of life is a "Sunday," a "prayer meeting," a "worship service."

Got home from Wisconsin and Don brought me supper in bed: fresh corn on the cob, tomatoes from Esther's garden, etc. We watched the news and then I went out in the big room to spend more time organizing my toys, all those twenty bags of puppets and each bag contains about ten puppets, surprises that children love. Each bag relates to a certain set of songs. I'll have to get rid of them; I almost cried. I've already gotten rid of quite a few of them by selling them out in our resale shop. We talked to Pete on the phone again. I promised him my "Trick Bag" cause he's planning to use puppets with children sometime. He's so good with kids. I guess he's a chip off the block. Phyllis was tickled with my gift of "Nitty Gritty Critty Band" puppets. Then we went to bed and made love!

(Surprised you, didn't I?)

Still can't get Jill on the phone. Hope all is well. Got the neatest letter from Holly today. Don and I were both crying as we read it. She's having a hard time facing my imminent death. So am I, but it's a reality. Holly, thanks for taking care of Tim, and giving us two wonderful grandsons.

I remember my times with little Bryan and the time he invited me to his class to sing. I was so proud to stand in front of his kindergarten class and was just prepared to introduce myself as Bryan's grandmother when suddenly a little voice from one of his classmates in the front row spoke up, and with a clear loud voice said, "You look old!"

"I am old," I said quickly, "'cause I'm Bryan's grandmother." I love kids.

I wish I could have handled our relationships better, Holly. I'm sorry. I just "freak out" over the perils of alcohol; it's so insidious. I love you guys so much. I have faith that you will live a happy life.

Maybe Co will call tonight. She said she would come home again and spend more time if we need her. Sylvia just called and talked an hour. She's so concerned that we have to sell our stuff. She said she bought all those puppets I had in the shop so we would know where they are...how thoughtful! Don and I are not attached to our things. We like to think our experience with the Reba Place commune helped mold our attitude toward earthly possessions. We had fun collecting, and now we're having fun distributing to someone else. We look at it like another adventure. People cannot understand us...really, do we have a choice? (The redness on my chest looks worse every day.) I'm just happy I can help organize it so the people that can use it will understand where the parts are. I remember when you kids would put on shows out in our garage and beg us to come out and watch. I was in the middle of a thousand things, but I so enjoyed watching you have fun being creative. Remember when Tim directed the "Miracle Worker" play when he was just fourteen; and in one of the wild scenes, he even used ketchup for blood? Don is snoring now so I'll watch TV. I love you guys so much tonight.

**"Let us then try what love will do,
For if people did once see we love,
Then we should soon find they would not harm us."**
- William Penn 1692

    We had such a fun day going "garaging." Imagine, we're going to sell our stuff soon and here we go to find more. We found some things for gifts and a few things we'll try to make some bucks; we call it gas money. We headed toward Palatine because Gerry Wayne told us about a new grocery store and it lived up to her billing. We didn't get much, but it was fun to see all the salads, fresh flowers, etc. We shared a soup and salad, took in a few more sales, and then at Don's suggestion went home. He gets tired of it sooner than I. I'm just glad he likes going with me.
    We practiced for an hour tonight, and I felt like I could have gone longer. I organized all my music stuff which I'll leave in the basement for anyone to share. We've been

hearing rumblings of meetings going on where we are not invited; I can't wait to hear what all the secrets are about. Talked to Jill and the family tonight; they seemed so happy.

Today started with lots of rain and then turned out to be a beautiful day. Don made his first apple pie and lots of apple sauce. I was very weak today so Don has been my gopher. He's so good to me. We took a drive around Woodstock tonight, stopped for D-Queen. Poor Don wanted a chocolate fudge sundae so bad, but he's trying so hard to get under 200 again, and just can't make it. I decided to take my sleeping pills early tonight because it's getting so hard to find any position that's comfortable. Good night, you're such a loved brood.

Just had a good night's sleep till 5:30 and then Don got up and made me breakfast in bed: orange slices, granola, wheat toast, coffee, and shark's cartilage...what's that, you say? We decided to try this as one more attempt to find a solution for cancer...300 tablets for $100.00, three a day. I'm a bit scared to start the day because of the lung aspiration at the ER. Esther said she'd be there. What a great lady she is. I hope I can be brave, but sometimes I say, "Who cares, I'm me!"

That reminds me of the card Esther gave me showing piglet holding Pooh Bear's hand as they walked out into the woods. Piglet said, "Pooh Bear, it's so hard to be brave when I'm such a small animal."

Esther and John have been our greatest friends. John was in elementary school with me in Harleysville, Pennsylvania, and then we hadn't seen them until they became part of Reba Place Fellowship in the late 1960's. Soon after we moved to Woodstock they bought a home there also. We've had so many fun times together, traveling to New Orleans one fall. One year on John's birthday we tied a big red bow around our worn-out El Camino truck, drove it over to their house and handed John the keys. Now they are the owners and we can use it whenever we want. Of course, since Esther is a nurse at the hospital, she is my most important health link to survival.

Don is out running. He just started that routine lately, grumbling all the while. He'd rather walk with me like we used to. My mind computes that memory often, just like we used to dream of growing old together and where we would live. Actually, I've realized most of my dreams, I guess, and feel very grateful, especially for the time Don has been able to be with me since he retired early in 1987. We didn't know at the time, of course, that I had cancer; now we look at that decision he made when he was just fifty-five as being such a milestone in our lives because of all the things we did together since then that would not have been possible otherwise.

The whole Russia chapter that really began in 1986 when Don wrote a letter to President Gorbachev. Actually, he wrote a letter to President Reagan, too, but only got a response from Gorbachev. I remember getting this strange-looking letter in the mail when Don was at school, and thinking it was just some third class mail I put in on the discard stack. As Don was leafing through that stack of "junk" mail, he suddenly shouted, "A letter from Gorbachev!" Of course, Don has all those memories to pine about if I'm gone.

Maybe my bum knee is related to my cancer, I never thought of that before. My shortness of breath just will not allow me to even walk for five minutes without real difficulty. Right now I feel like getting out of bed and practicing all my instruments. That is my greatest job, but I love to do it best when no one is here. It is a real moment of worship for me.

I start with the piano, then to the other strings for awhile...banjo, guitar, dulcimer, just enough mandolin to get by, my little psaltry, then the five-stringed instrument that Dean brought back to me from Yugoslavia, some recorder music, and then I go to my bag of puppets, imagining that there are lots of kids in front of me. See, I have loads of joy yet....

Music was her passion. She was determined to include a variety of instruments in her shows. Sometimes I balked at carrying all those suitcases; now I think how selfish of me! She was proficient in guitar, but most other instruments were used for interest, including harp, violin, accordion, recorder, uke, piano, organ, and string bass. She even took a few lessons on the tenor sax so she could entertain with "When the Saints Go Marching In."

Here comes Don, puffing, and said, "It's still not fun." Vic and Marie Stoltzfus, president of Goshen College, just called and reminded us of the Stoltzfus reunion that we missed and to invite themselves to visit us soon. That is Don's mother's side of the family. Vic is Don's first cousin. The Stoltzfus clan emigrated from the Palatinate in Germany in the late eighteenth century, I believe.

When we lived in Goshen, 1956-58, there were four men first cousins enrolled in college at the same time: Vic and Bryan Stoltzfus, Richard Metzler, and Don, all married. We would all get together occasionally for good times. Often Vic and Marie would baby-sit our three oldest kids if we wanted to get out for the evening.

Sherry Steffen from Wisconsin called and said she was here visiting friends and stopped in to see me three times, but I wasn't home. Now she wonders whether she could sneak by before returning home. While talking on the phone to her, I cried and cried 'cause my memories of ten years ago returned. I used to listen to her terrible stories of being mistreated by her husband at the time. She was one of my special guitar students. Now she wants to be here for me. Her life is still tough because her new husband can't get along with her own kids. Are all husbands that way, she wonders? I told her, "I just can't handle anymore company now; let's just talk on the phone." See, I'm honest enough to say "No" sometimes. She had a friend who wanted to meet me, but being the great person she is, she understood perfectly that now was not the right time. Then she told me of another coincidence. She is good friends of a Kingston Trio groupie who travels to Vegas and other places with Sherry to hear them. What a surprise to Sherry when this friend said, "Of course, I know Eunice Mast. I was in her home with the Kingston Trio five years ago."

Another great day...waited till 9:00 p.m. to hear from the doctor about aspirating my lungs. Just then Marian called again and is begging God to heal me. I pray "Amen" and hope she has healing power through prayer that I don't seem to have. All I can honestly pray is, "Thank you, God. I've had such a good life and family and, Lord, you know I'd love to be healed." Then Odette Musial called and wanted to visit for the first time since her husband died of lung and brain cancer the past winter while we were in California. She let it all hang out; we cried and laughed.

While she was here a group from Plow Creek Fellowship, near Tiskilwa, Illinois, who are friends from the Reba Place days, came to visit. Don showed the Begleys around while I was with Odette. Later that evening we went for a drive and out for dinner in McHenry. When we got home we decided to practice before settling in, but we barely got started before we were interrupted five times. A call from Millers in Canada ended our practice session. Louise Miller is so weak from her Parkinson's that they were announcing they couldn't come to the special September celebration...did I talk about that yet? Later I guess. We all ended up crying on the phone remembering the great times we had in Goshen in 1956-57 as we sought to form a church true to the spirit of Jesus. John was Professor of Old Testament at the seminary in those days. Our life with Millers continued at the Reba Place Fellowship in 1957 in Evanston, Illinois. Now Louise and I are nearing the end.

No sooner did she hang up than Esther was on the phone telling me how much she loves me. Wow, how can I absorb all this love. I told Esther that I'll be meeting her in the morning in the ER according to Dr. Lynd. Then I learned from Letty that a friend is hurt because she wasn't invited to the birthday party we had for Hackmans. Sometimes I don't cover all bases. Sorry!

Before settling in for the night, Tim called to say "Hello" and wanted to know how I was feeling. He sounded so good. Holly got her new job; Bryan always loves to say "I love you, Grandma"; what a neat kid. Thank you, God, for this family; I'll hate to leave them. Don is watching the ballgame on TV. He has the sound down so low because he knows I can't care for football, or is it baseball, I don't even know the difference. My poor husband is so good to me. Dean called and brought me up-to-date on the kids. Dean, I hope you make them take music instruments, too. Kids have to be introduced to these things even though they resist it at first. Later they'll thank you for it. I was the "pusher" in our family; Don didn't have the patience to put up with lackluster practices.

I am so proud that I'm keeping up with this diary. I have no idea if it's interesting to anyone but it better be! It ain't easy to do. Don and I are reading this new cancer treatment book on shark's cartilage. So many of our friends are encouraging us to take this or that treatment. Don's sister, Beula, followed many special diets for her cancer, and died three years later. I decided not to go that route; my hunch is that with my advanced stage of cancer, I have about three years and that's it, regardless what I take.

Eunice's cancer was diagnosed in July 1991 already in stage 4, advanced. She died thirty months later. Clyde and Kathy Weaver lived near us in Elgin and had been relating to us over the last several years. Kathy was diagnosed with cancer about the same time as Eunice, but Kathy was convinced to stay with the "holistic" approach. Clyde died in April 1994 of a heart attack, and Kathy died in June 1994. Eunice was on KM, a potassium mineral supplement for awhile, too, but she felt her body was under so much strain with all the treatments that she resorted to the doctor's scientific advice of chemo. Another friend wondered whether we would be open to her "Scientology" approach. And yet another friend tried to get her interested in biofeedback, meditation, and mind/body healing. It was amazing the many different ideas for healing we encountered. But, true to form, Eunice had no interest in complicated cures. She wanted to keep laughing, playing guitar and singing, and eating as long as she was alive, and she was enjoying all of those things up until a week or so before she died.

I want to just be sensible: "Eat dessert first, cause life is short"...."Carpe diem," seize the day, as Colleen used to tell me. She wrote it in large letters on the chalkboard. I feel like I have it all right now; I don't want to die very soon, but don't pity me or you if I do. Make a difference in this world and be proud of yourself. "Yin and yang" is the balance of everything in life. I saw that on TV tonight about the ancient Chinese philosophy.

It's 10:00 and just time for one more phone call. It was Bill Shaw wanting to talk to Don about inviting Peter, Paul, and Mary along on the Russian trip summer of

1994. Don has been working with some agents of musicians to help Bill locate some good singers for the proposed trip.

---

*"Only when we are no longer afraid
do we begin to live in every experience,
painful or joyous;
to live in gratitude for every moment,
to live abundantly."*
- *Dorothy Thompson*

Tuesday morning 6:45...this is it! I'm not emotionally ready for this aspiration, but I know that Esther will be there and Dr. Lynd is a great surgeon. There she was waiting for me, plus two nurses that I worked with when I had been a volunteer in ER. I knew I was in trouble when one of the nurses asked, "Did you ever have this done before?"

When I said, "No," they exchanged nervous glances. That was enough for me. I braced myself and tried to stay calm. The doctor placed my head on a pillow on the metal cart while the nurses held me down. "I'm not going anywhere," I tried to assure them.

"We're only doing this for you because you're so special," said one....(yeh, right!) I was working hard not to wince at the pain. Two hours later and two x-rays, they had drained a quart of fluid, and now I'm supposed to be better?

Don was waiting for me and we went out for breakfast. I began thinking of all the individuals I met either at the therapy sessions, doctor's office, etc., that came there alone and had to leave alone because they didn't have a husband or child to grieve with them. I'm a lucky person. I wonder if those acquaintances I met in passing are still living. Like ships passing in the night, I thought. I meet someone with great pain and anxiety, and just like that they're gone.

Don and I played some cards, but of course, I'm very sore where the tube was placed in my body. Amazing I still wanted to practice, so we spent some time singing until Jerry Paulson came and wanted to talk to us about the upcoming committee gathering tomorrow at our house. It still wasn't a certainty that we would have the Singalong at our house after we leave because we hadn't found someone to rent our place who would willingly open their home for a group of 200 every first Saturday of the month. Would you? The committee was not prepared to rent the house just to have the singing once a month. "What to do?" as the Nikitins used to say in Russian when they faced perplexing problems. Jerry warned us that many people were having a very tough time accepting the end of the Masthouse Singalong, much less my death! Great!! Don and I have worked through this with ourselves; now we have to help others work through it, too.

Eunice is referring to a decision I made to designate the September Singalong a tribute to Eunice and all the music she brought to this community through guitar lessons, albeit therapy sessions sometimes. Many of our friends knew that we were going to sell our things and possibly move to California with our kids later this fall. So we spread the word that there would be changes.

While we were talking with Jerry, Val Gitlin and Jan Marsh came to pick me up for lunch at the Woodstock Country Club. We had great conversation, that is, they did, because I wanted to save my breath and stay out of the talking as much as I could. They wanted to know about our leaving, etc. I explained our plans for a sale. What a relief to know that Val, Joyce, and Marian volunteered to price all the stuff, beginning the first day after the September Singalong; they figured it would take about two weeks to do it all. What a job! I'm so happy because I trust their judgment on the pricing.

Marian had some trouble with it because while she's praying for my recovery it looks as though we're giving up if we sell. She is so convinced of a concept of healing I can't fathom. Don and I had invited our kids to choose one expensive object from our collection, and many mementos that we would keep for them.

Don and I practiced again, more eating and sorting music. Then at 10:00, this day that began in the ER, this tired woman put her poor old body down.

"A personal story about a special person....

From the time that I was a very young woman, I felt as though Adam and Eve were just part of a creation myth. But when I became a Baha'í, I learned that Baha'u'lláh spoke of Adam as the first messenger of God. And as is the nature of faith, because I believed in Baha'u'lláh, I grew to believe in Adam, too. Then not too many months ago a group of scientists announced that they had proven, through their DNA research, that all women were descendants of one woman— the mother of the races, so to speak. Now I had an Eve for Adam. As a woman, and a mother, I got to wondering what Eve would have been like. If she were alive today, I think that she would have a spiritual furnace burning inside of her, burning so strongly that it would attract souls to her, without them even knowing why. She would be very connected to the earth, living the rhythms of womanhood through courtship, marriage, child birth and motherhood, always willing to adapt to the new roles her life required. And she would be endowed with virtues which she would balance to work for her. She would be honest herself, and trusting of others, generous and imminently practical, friendly, intelligent, creative and willing to accept the authority of God, her own creator. She would set high moral standards for herself, and expect those around her to respect these standards. And above all, she would find much to celebrate in this life on earth. She would celebrate through her talents, and encourage others to find their talents as artists, musicians, or poets.

She would know that her life here on earth was important to her eternal life, and would not waste it. And when she realized that she would no longer be part of this physical reality, she would let that go, too, with grace.

As you can clearly see, this picture of ideal womanhood—spiritual, creative, virtuous, practical, and loving—sounds like a myth, too. But you can also see that it was, in reality, fulfilled in the life of Eunice.   - Laurie Rosenfield

---

Jill wrote a lovely letter today. Time to listen to a few words from Oprah. Don went for some groceries for breakfast and then we'll sit on the deck and start the day. The pills worked again last night. I slept till 8:00 a.m., still with some pain from the operation. The morning ritual starts with a dressing change on my groshong catheter, which is an implant catheter in my chest that allows easier blood withdrawal and can later also be used for morphine injection; what a life! Now I'll wait for Nurse Mary. She always allows me plenty of time to share any feelings. Don just called, "Breakfast on the deck."

Esther came later on and brought us a treat and we talked and talked. She is so precious to me. The committee is meeting in our room right now, talking about the future of the Singalong, and asked us if we would mind not being part of the meeting till they call us. It's been almost two hours; what is going on?

Fred Boger came and made two beautiful bouquets today, one for the porch and one for the room; bless his heart. He's a seventish man who loves the Singalong and is determined to see it continue somewhere. Don and I are looking favorably to having it continue here. We had been a bit unsure, not knowing yet who might be living here. When Letty was here today to give us some sweets, we shared the idea with her about the Singalong future without us. She has been so good to us and we want her to be happy. It made me feel good to know that she was pleased with the idea. She is so devastated about my illness, saying she would rather take my sickness herself. Doesn't that sound like a Biblical example of love?

Today the first letter I opened was from Joanna Lehman, one of our friends from Reba Place in Evanston. The letter started, "Eunice, I'm writing to you to say 'Good-bye' etc...." I burst out crying and Don helped me get over it. I don't want to say "Good-bye" to people yet. The letter was so warm, saying how much I meant to her while we were part of the fledgling commune. She always seemed to idolize me too much. She also has breast cancer, but in an earlier stage.

Colleen called a little bit ago and she helped us come to terms with the handling of our stuff. You kids have all been so good about it; I don't feel any greediness which happens so often.

"Nothing is worth more than this day." - *Goethe*

Some new signs in my mouth of soreness; also I had to take some nausea pills for the chemotherapy today. Mom called today and seems at peace with my situation. Here they are in their upper eighties, and I'm floundering.

A few from the committee have knocked on the door and want to share with us the results of the meeting. The upshot is that they want to continue the Singalongs as is, and they will pay us for the things that remain in the music room. They will take all responsibility for the operation of the event, including cleaning, etc. They will also pay us $100 per Singalong night to cover utilities and the use of the room. In addition, they are organizing a benefit in November to help us buy an RV. This benefit will be an all-day music event that will draw on the best folk artists in the Chicago area. Their love seems to have no bounds; they want us to not lift a finger in preparation. ....Sure!

August 23, 1993: Today Don and I practiced a lot. I feel so good...so we'll make hay while the sun shines. Later we decided to run away for awhile. Don said I should get anything I wanted for my birthday. We ended up at the Kenosha outlet store, what fun! Don and I cried almost the whole way there. At times the whole payload just overwhelms us and we have to release. I spent a lot of time at the Dollar store then gave the bag to Don while I continued my shopping delight. Don stretched out in the van for two hours till I got my fill. Thanks so much, Peter, for the van; it has been my joy in these last days. I found my birthday gift from Don. (He tells me to buy it; that way I'll get what I want. I like that.) I bought the most beautiful nightwear I could find so I'll have something nice when I need to be in bed "at the end." I guess that sounds a little maudlin, but I just want to be prepared; it's realistic. We spent a lot of time tonight packing books and other stuff to give to the kids; I hope they like it.

That first frantic month following my mastectomy in July 1991 flashes before me so often. The one joy of that month was when Peter handed over the money to buy our '88 Chevy van. Our first trip was to the Milwaukee clinic.

The head of the oncology department treated us very unprofessionally when he learned we wanted to get a second opinion from Mayo clinic. "I thought you would welcome our concern about treatment if you are a professional doctor who cares. This is my body that has cancer," I blurted out to him amidst tears.

It was an unpleasant scene. That's the day we returned home to find the card from Pete Seeger saying he wanted to stop in to see our Singalong when he comes to Wisconsin in November. That was the emotional boost Eunice needed. I answered Pete immediately and we prepared for the big event. As November approached the excitement grew. Then an unexpected phone call from the Nikitins in Moscow. They said they were coming to the states in November and wondered whether they could visit us. My wheels started spinning because I knew they had never met Pete. He was their American idol since the days they heard him at Moscow University in the '60's.

Well, we had the Mother of all Singalongs in November with Nikitins and Pete on stage with us, and Eunice was ecstatic. We drove to Madison to pick up Pete and on the drive to Woodstock I asked Pete to sit in back with Eunice. She shared her music upbringing, her bout with cancer, her love of life, then she prodded him with questions. "Do you like people taking pictures of you?" she asked. "Only when I don't know it," Pete said. There upon she whipped out the little Kodak and snapped a picture of him at her side.

I feel super this morning. My chest is still very red and itchy. It's scary cause the cancer is so noticeable with lots of lumps under the skin all around my chest wall; it gets worse every day, but I feel great today. The sleeping pills didn't work last night, so I read more of the Klondike book. Maybe it's because I ate lots of chocolate last night; that's it, I'm sure.

I felt like cooking today: bread made out of stale cereal and nuts, raisins; pickled beet eggs. John Aiello, our plumber, keeps bringing me eggs. He said, "They'll last one or two years in the frig." I'm afraid he meant it.

I made dolmas which is a rice-meat-herb mix that I wrap in my homegrown blanched Swiss chard, then pour seasoned vinegar on it, then a huge fresh Hackman tomato salad, two big corn meal tamale pies, cheese garlic dip, etc. Well, at 7:30 we have a small group here for a party including Hans and Sherry. I have a feeling they're having troubles. I'd just crave to say, "Let's talk it out." I hope they get some professional help; we all need help at times when we have to live with another human. It's better not to waste precious time arguing about things if someone can help you. Wetzels were here so the four of us stayed up till midnight talking.

Next morning Sherry asked to borrow some video tapes I had ordered to give to our children. They are marriage self-help tapes that are wonderful. I felt good knowing that they want to use them as they look forward to getting married sometime in 1994. I have the feeling I will be in another world for that event, but I'll watch from above, Hans and Sherry. Building relationships is not easy. I truly believe that living at Reba Place helped Don and me through our early years. You must be honest and want help.

Yesterday Don showed his "wart"; I think he only has one. While we were practicing he made the same mistake that he makes so frequently in a song, but he refuses to write it down so that he can learn. He is so stubborn sometimes. I used to pout till I got my way, but now I accept that for some strange reason he has to go through that frustration and I'll go through it with him and never get mad about it again. He has so many good qualities to rejoice about that I won't let that one get me down.

Around noon, Susan Urban and Phil Cooper showed up for a spontaneous lunch 'cause she wanted to finish shooting some more pictures for her video on the Masthouse. She's a professional photographer as well as a singer. I can't wait to see the video. I feel like a celebrity these days, spoiled rotten.

Later we needed to get away again so we headed for the Rockford mall where I did some more "70% off" shopping. Each time I do this I think maybe this is the last shopping spree I'll do in my whole lifetime; it gives me an eerie feeling. Just you wait till it's your turn. I got a few neat clothes and a nice black silk shirt for Don. (See, I get new clothes sometimes; it's not as much fun as finding brand names at a used shop for a quarter.)

When I got home, I was ready to work again. Don cleaned and I practiced instruments. My life is so rich; why does it have to end? Again I couldn't sleep till 3:00 a.m., then took my pills and slept till Don brought me a late breakfast in bed.

We had lunch on the deck, the "Riviera" we call it. We love to sit there and look over the garden and flowers and talk about the joys of living. That's the title of a song I've been learning. It's strange to think we won't be living here very long anymore, yet I'm glad to look forward to better things. Amy came this morning and we talked and enjoyed the bubbles I keep in a small container on the deck. The magic of bubbles is so soothing and fun.

I'm gonna get busy now and clean up the kitchen. Don just came in for a kiss; he needs to be pampered a little. Someone had just called and wondered whether we know how much trouble we're causing people just because we're moving; he even seemed a little irritated. Brother! We had lunch with Hans, dinner with Hackmans, and tomorrow a party with Steve and Sylvia.

We had so much fun with Hackmans. One of the laughs on me was my memory of the time years ago when I was asked to perform for the ladies' auxiliary luncheon. Now these are the fancy ladies. Well, I never turn down an invitation to sing. Each month a guest performer provides music while the ladies can have their glasses filled and talk to each other about their new wardrobes prior to the business meeting. It is a difficult job to try to entertain a loud group of drinkers. I had dressed casually, but appropriately I thought, for the event with long flowing skirt purchased recently at the "Second Chance" store in town. Who knows, I thought, maybe my dress once belonged to one of these fine ladies. I was wearing my matching blue/black heeled shoes, and a smile, always. I was moving gaily around the room with no designated stage, kicking up my heels and singing at the top of my lungs.

A half hour later I took my seat as the group came to order and I nervously fidgeted around, hoping I had entertained properly. When to my amazement as I lifted one leg on top of the other, I noticed my shoes were not a pair. I will never know, and I didn't ask if any of the ladies ever noticed.

I need to watch TV....

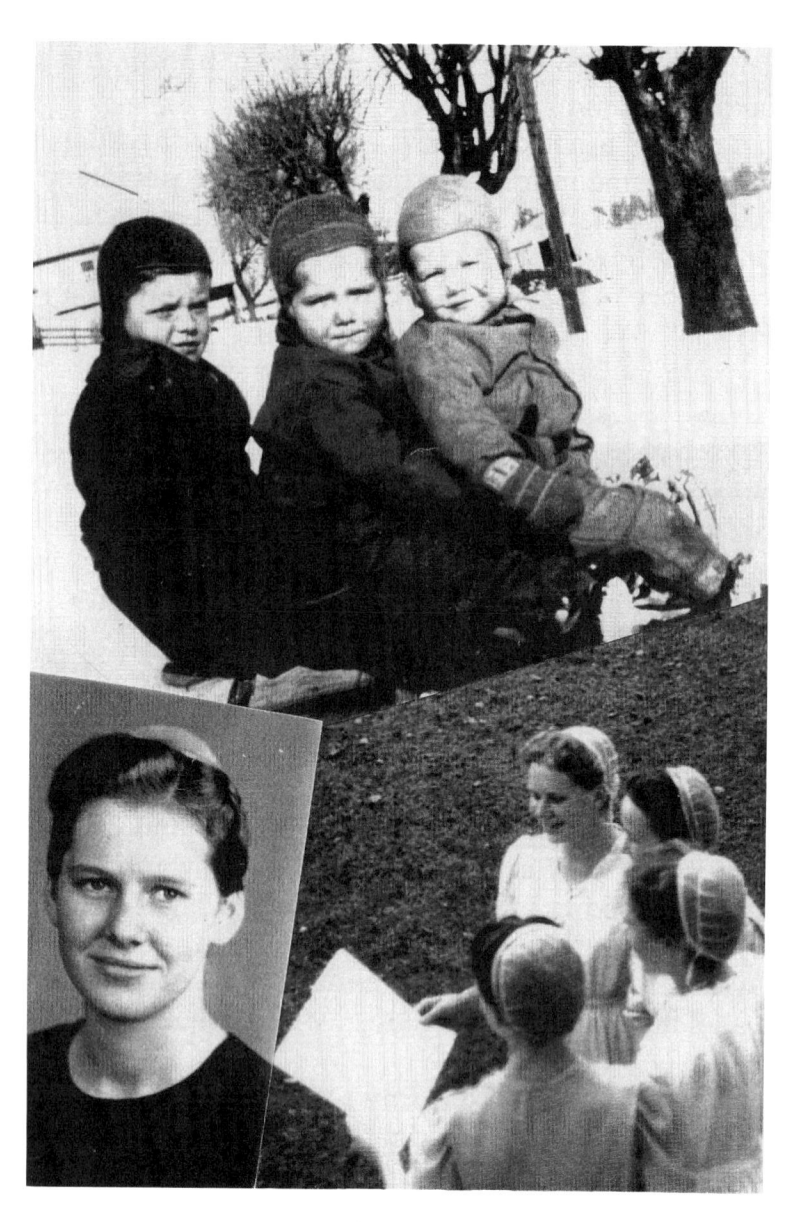

Top: Eunice (right) with her brother John (left) and sister Lois (middle). **Bottom left:** Eunice's 1951 graduation picture from Eastern Mennonite High School, Harrisonburg, Virginia. **Bottom right:** Eunice singing in a ladies' quartet.

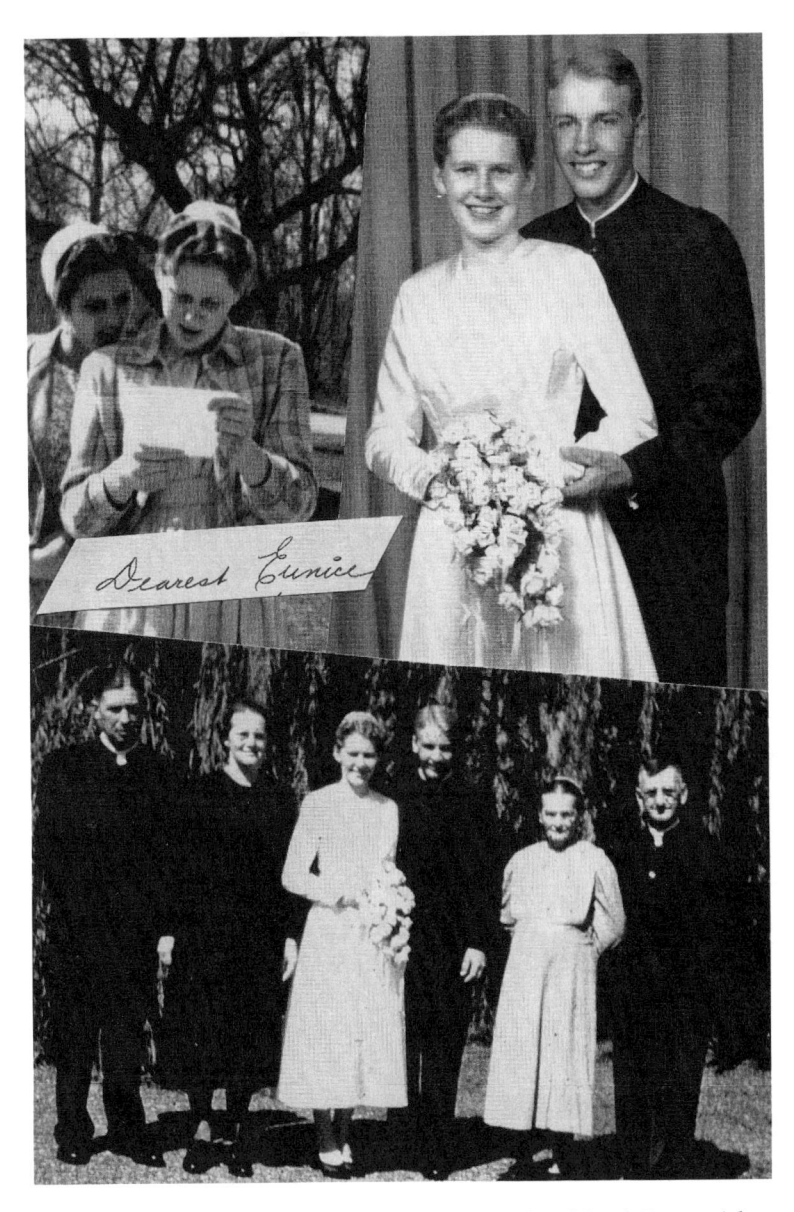

Top left: *Eunice reading a letter from her boyfriend Don with a friend peering over her shoulder. ("Dearest Eunice" is Don's handwriting at that time.)* ***Top right:*** *Don and Eunice on their wedding day, September 6, 1952.* ***Bottom:*** *Don and Eunice (center) on their wedding day with both parents, Henry and Susan Ruth and Mamie and David Mast.*

Not what we give, but what we share

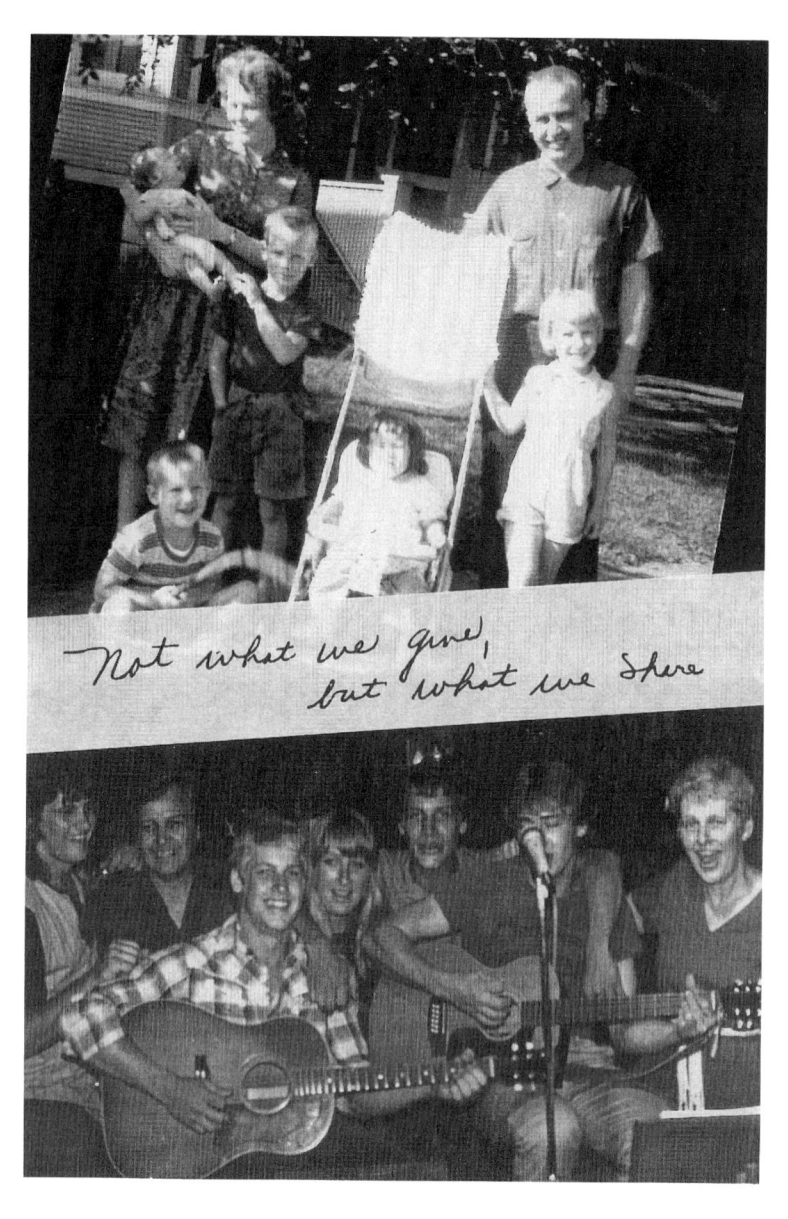

Top: Eunice and Don and their young family in front of their house at Reba Place. (Photograph shows five children. Hans was not yet born.) **Bottom:** Don and Eunice and their children (except Jill) enjoying "sharing" their music together. **Center quote:** This is Eunice's handwriting, taken from a poem by James Russell Lowell (1819-1891).

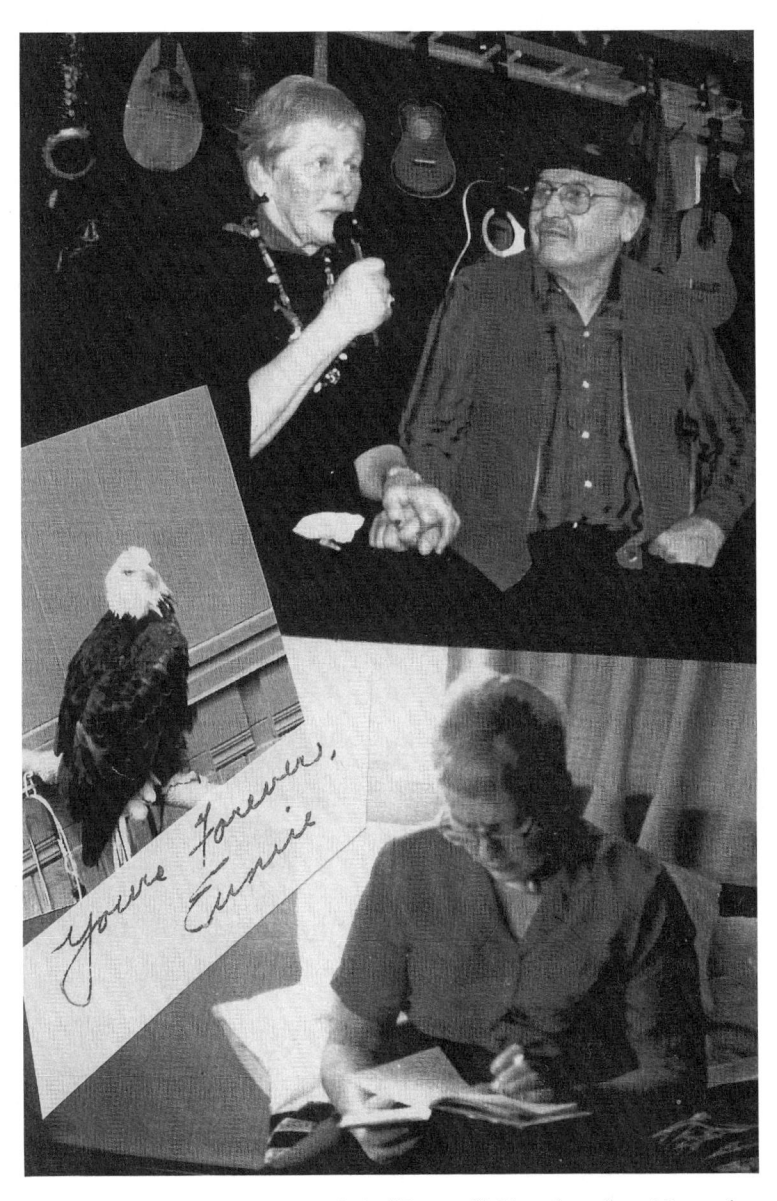

Top: *Eunice participating in their "Farewell Singalong" on November 6, 1993, at Masthouse while she holds Don's hand for support. Photo by R. W. Block.* ***Center:*** *Eunice's fascination with eagles even served as a symbol to her own impending flight.* ***Bottom:*** *Eunice writing in her journal at the Vancouver Hotel. Her own handwriting, "Yours forever, Eunice," was taken from a letter to Don and is symbolic of her living on through this book.*

My mind often drifts back to childhood, especially when I think of one of my favorite songs, "Music in My Mother's House," written by Stuart Stotts. I can't remember if I already wrote about it. This past July, Don and I hosted the Midwest Song Writer's Assembly. Some thirty people gathered from Illinois. Wisconsin, Kansas, and other parts to share their new songs and offer hints on songwriting. That's where I first met Stuart. The last night of the gathering we sang around the circle, each leading a favorite song. Stuart was last and we all sang with him "Music in My Mother's House." What a grand feeling, but I sensed we weren't quite finished so I grabbed my accordion and said, "Any of you that still have an ounce of energy, follow me around the room." After playing a Russian dance tune, I asked everyone to put hands on another's shoulder and sing "Amazing Grace." Lots of tears flowed freely. No one wanted the precious weekend of sharing music and ideas to end. Stuart said he went off to a corner and wrote this song when everyone was saying "Good-byes":

> "We will dance at midnight
> When the last song has been sung;
> Hand in hand in the lamplight with the old,
> The departed, and the young.
>
> Round the room, past the couches
> Where guitars and drums are hung;
> Music heals what it touches
> When the last song has been sung.
>
> As we stand in the silence
> There's a word on every tongue;
> We will bring these words home with us
> When the last song has been sung."

I'm behind in writing. I slept well last night; sleeping pills worked again. Don and I had another good talk; I can't believe how well I feel today. I barely got ready in time for Nurse Mary who came to work on my chemo hookup. While she was flushing my groshong catheter I suddenly fainted; that's the first that happened. Later some ladies came to take me to Lake Geneva for my birthday party, August 25; I'm sixty today. What a time we had and an elegant meal, interrupted by the playing of "Happy Birthday" by the pianist while the room full of patrons sang and cheered, then gifts. You see how I'm spoiled? Don made a video of me with the puppets that I want to give to Peter who would be an ideal puppeteer since he's so good with kids.

This morning two huge plants were delivered to the door from our son Hans and my sister Carolyn. My house looks like a greenhouse; I feel so loved. Yesterday during the luncheon with the ladies I had a fit of uncontrollable tears because I knew this was my last. I find myself in that frame often, "It is my last." My chest is so tight with tumors; redness continues to spread down my stomach, although I feel so good right now. So many people are praying; what does it mean? "Thank you, God," is all I can say. My brother John just called reminding us of their arrival at O'Hare on Saturday.

Did I tell you he and Roma are coming to film the big Celebration Singalong on Saturday? He is a film producer, and I am honored that he would break his busy schedule to come out here with his equipment. I call it my "wake" The committee is coming now for a meeting. We had a party, of course, discussed the November benefit being planned. As crazy at it may sound we went with the Francois' to a restaurant for cheeseburgers after the party; I know it's a way to share thoughts as much as to eat. They told us they had just gotten back from a concert in Milwaukee where they had talked with the Kingston Trio. The Trio had remembered visiting with us a few years back and wondered how we were doing. Toshi Seeger, Pete's wife, wrote this week discussing the proposed Russian trip and offered some suggestions of singers since Pete will not be able to join us after all. She wondered about my cancer and mentioned that Pete's sister had just died of cancer.

"I share with you the agony of your grief,
The anguish of your heart finds echo in my own.
I know I cannot enter all you feel
Nor bear with you the burden of your pain;
I can but offer what my love does give:
The strength of caring;
The warmth of one who seeks to understand,
The silent storm-swept barrenness of so great a loss
This I do in quiet ways that on your lonely path
You may not walk alone."
                                                    - *Howard Thurman*

I just changed the dressing on my groshong; Don is snoring so I'll cuddle beside him for awhile and watch TV. I can't find my sleeping pills so I'll probably stay awake all night. Peter just called; he didn't even know it was my birthday. He seems so happy even though he's so vulnerable about his work because people take advantage of his kindness and he often underestimates a job. He hires laborers from Tia Juana and pays them more than he keeps for himself. Oh well, I guess that's what we've been teaching, but now it doesn't seem fair.

Twila and Sharon from Pennsylvania, Don's nieces, just called about their visit here in September to help us with our sale. What neat people. Sue Bernstein from Evanston wants to spend a couple hours visiting. I was feeling absolutely lousy when Don called me to the deck. He wanted to read a letter he had prepared to send to our mailing list about our upcoming sale, my health etc. I burst into tears and poor Don didn't know what to do. It was a nice letter.

I was just unprepared again. So he held me and we cried together for five minutes. Then I pushed myself away and said, "Now that's enough, I'm done. Let's get to work!" When I grumbled about my nausea, Don reminded me to get my pills. I promised myself not to grumble cause I hate taking those pills. Just then a bell went off in my head. Listen to this story.

I remembered the marijuana joints that Dean left with me when he visited last summer. "Just in case," he said, "if it really gets uncomfortable, try it." I couldn't think of a more appropriate time. I ran to the drawer, got some matches, and was ready for business. Some health digests have recommended marijuana would relieve nausea. Don's lying on the floor in awe as I sit on his Father's Day chair trying my darndest to smoke. I tried every which way to get the thing lit and Don was rolling on the floor laughing hysterically watching me puffing and blowing streams of blue smoke. It was not ten minutes and the phone started ringing, and guess who it was. It was Mom, wondering how I was and what I was doing. She's so worried anyway that I won't get in the "Pearly gates" and here I am puffing a joint, trying to recover from a fit of laughter; Don was certainly no help rolling in the corner, not believing. I've never been happier that phone lines are still not visual. After a few pleasantries she reads me a poem that Lois sent her about memory loss. It was a funny poem, but the real funny part was that Mom was laughing so hard she couldn't read it. So we both ended up laughing and laughing. Wow, if humor heals the body, I should never have gotten sick. Mom has been so helpful in trying to lift my spirits.

Also, Carol came with her child who was vomiting because of a virus. I'm so nervous because of germs around me, but I didn't have the nerve to tell her to leave.

I just looked over my writing and noticed how poorly I write, but I don't care; I just want people to know what life is like with cancer. And to think, it's not present in my family, just in Don's. We think the environment is the cause, but what. Please, someone find the answer. Ken Marsh, bless his heart, has established a foundation of scientists who are trying to track it down.

Today I was sitting at my "throne," my stool at the kitchen bar, waiting for the doctor to call to confirm the date of the next batch of chemo treatments when I noticed the mail just arrived and here was my favorite magazine, *Sing Out*. I opened to the index to find out if there were any special songs and immediately saw a title I had never seen before, "The Joy of Living" by Ewan McColl.

Ewan is married to Peggy Seeger, Pete Seeger's sister. The title already was a winner and I quickly ran for my guitar to pick out the tune and words. He wrote it as a farewell to the world and all the people he loved, because he was dying of cancer.

Eunice and I changed some of the words to fit her own cancer condition. The song was dear to her and she had practically learned it before she died. She was prepared to sing it at the November Singalong, but she was afraid the emotion of the hour would be too much....She continues.

That song sums it up real good for me. In spite of the fact that I can hardly write this for the tears in my eyes, half or more are shed because of the joy and peace I'm blessed with. Thank you, God. I'm no dummy. I know how blest I've been with such a wonderful family, starting with parents, brother, and sisters, to the best husband anyone could hope for, down to six wonderful children. We'll overlook the tough years; eight very special grandchildren. And then I think of all the friends and people who have touched my life. No one could have asked for more. I'm busy, which makes life exciting. I better go clean the frig cause Don just made a mess spilling a dish of redbeet eggs. I'm not going to grumble though, 'cause Lord knows what he's going to have to do with me yet. By the way, I'm not nauseated anymore; maybe that "weed" worked! Maybe I should try again, or perhaps it was the laughter, praise the Lord.

Gerry just stopped in and brought me a copy of *The New York Times*. The cover has a picture of a model who wants to make a statement about breast cancer, and so she has her right breast exposed showing the mastectomy. It's strange, gruesome!

Don is making some folders with hymns to be sung by our family at the Singalong. I expect there will be about twelve of my family and in-laws here. There are times I feel sad that my own children were not brought up in a normal Mennonite Church so they could have learned these beautiful hymns, but there are trade-offs. Really I have never regretted the path we took over the last forty years since leaving the safe confines of our church in Pennsylvania.

These glorious twenty-two years in Woodstock we have been surrounded by a loving spiritual community of people who nurture one another, crossing all cultural and religious lines: we are Bahai, Mennonite, Friends,

Unitarians, Evangelicals, Catholics, and who knows what else, no one asks, cause it doesn't matter. As I read the letters of caring, I get strength to ride the tide. I am so moved by the compassionate God that has been available to all these varied faiths throughout the world; it makes me embarrassed to get hung up on trivia.

> **"A butterfly lights beside us like a sunbeam,**
> **And for a brief moment**
> **Its glory and beauty belong to our world.**
> **But then it flies on again,**
> **And though we wish it could have stayed,**
> **We feel so lucky to have seen it."**
> *- Unknown*

Now I'm sitting in the doctor's office waiting for her to tell me if the cancer has spread. Dr. Ritzman is helpful, but she is so unreachable; when I really need her, she is unavailable. The question is, "Should I discontinue taking chemo and try another treatment like 'taxol', the new drug that is receiving a lot of attention?" Don's niece, Bernie, was taking it and decided to discontinue because of very unpleasant side effects. I'll wait to decide till after the Singalong. I'd rather feel better and die several months earlier. Sunday is my last children's program. That will be another crisis; my dear puppets that gave me so much pleasure. Then Monday the ladies are going to start pricing all our items for sale. I've already picked out the things I'm going to give the kids: six large suitcases full of stuff.

Two days till the Singalong. I've been feeling super these days; I hope it lasts through Saturday. I've been wined and dined so often. Today we decided to lock the door when we practiced so we wouldn't be interrupted so often. Bopparts took us out to eat in the evening, then the committee met once more to go over details before announcing the news to the Singalong crowd.

Becky Seip just wrote us a wonderful letter about her sadness of our leaving and a cute tear-jerker poem. I was so touched about her poem that I called her at work and impulsively asked her whether she wanted to live in our basement apartment and help take care of the place. She excitedly said, "Sure."

Woops! I don't have all the fixtures to dress my groshong so Don had to call Caremark. Last night we went to a neat restaurant in Greek town, all the trimmings with cake and ice cream.

Don plays volleyball each Thursday night with his friends in Evanston. He's reluctant to leave me, but I need time by myself, too. The phone keeps ringing; I think we have over sixty people who have signed up to perform Saturday night.

I think of the grandkids so often. We have eight now. They are all in California. For the past six years we have spent the winters with them. Those are precious memories with my song bags, puppets, and the kids. There goes the doorbell and the phone. When will we get our RV and get out of here?

Don just brought me oatmeal, sweet rolls, juice, and coffee. Now to a TV show for a mind settling. Whew! I'm in an unusual state of mind, one minute laughing and the next minute crying. Just to give you an idea, this morning, September 6, 1993, is our forty-first wedding anniversary. I decided to go over to Letty's to cheer her up because I knew she'd be having a hard time when the ladies start to price our things for the estate sale in two weeks. Just as she was coming to the door, I broke out in uncontrollable tears. We hugged and cried together.

One Week Later... How can I review the Singalong? I'll try to make it brief. There must have been over 400 people here. We picked up John and Roma at the airport on Saturday morning and I was bubbling all over. I had to sit through that whole evening with Don at my side, squeezing my hand and handing me hankies. The gift of friends I've too often taken for granted. By the way, this September 1993 Singalong is going to be on a video that you can own. It took the grace of God to absorb all the love, but what a remarkable experience!

During the evening, those who had no song to share could just come to the mike if they had something to tell me. We passed out hankies, threw teddy bears left and right, cried, kissed, and loved, a celebration I will never forget. Thank you, Don, for the idea and your constant support.

Family and guests are gone; the house is empty and quiet. The songs have been sung and I return to the world of cancer. That's my world. People can pray with me, rejoice with me, sing with me, but it's still my world. I have to "walk it by myself."

Now the sale! We've decided that we will convert the garage next door to our apartment, "the nest." That will be Don's home when I take wings. We have a lot of things already sorted: items for the kids, other things for the RV, essential things to the nest, most things to be sold which the ladies have started working on. What a relief to have Val, Marian, and Joyce carry the load of the sale.

The effect of the chemo is working on me now. I cried most of one day while everyone was working 'cause I alone can feel the seriousness of my cancer. My chest is very tight and hard and it's getting increasingly harder to breathe. I cry so easily because I'm weak. What I'd do without Don, I don't know. He's running around here from one person to the next who needs information. He's so strong and loving! I didn't sleep much last night even with my pills. The pain in my chest is much stronger and I get pretty depressed. I try to calm myself by centering on God and love; and it works.

Today I wrote lots of letters and stayed out of the "fray." Yesterday I made bread and potato cheeses, corn soup. Don said the ladies are finished pricing our sale items; they've been working steady for a week.

I'll take a nap....

Much Later. This is truly the first day for possibly months that I am relaxed and unpressured. But remember all that pressure was probably my lifesaver from depression and anxiety. It was mostly fun, exciting stuff. Don took over the sale: handing out numbers at 5:30 a.m., admitting twenty-five at a time beginning at 7:00, assigning helpers to collect money at the rear doors, handling hurt feelings, etc. Then a week later we had an auction, and any remaining items we either gave away or had a... guess what, "garage sale." Now I'm tired of sales.

The October Singalong came and went. Becky Seip moved into the basement, and wanted me to teach her how to bake bread so that she will take over that chore for the Singalongs.

Twila and Sharon were here and helped immensely with the sale; they've now gone home. Presently Dan Bumstead, Don's nephew, and wife Regina are here with their three kids helping to convert the garage into our "nest." I can't wait to get settled again, but I'm not frustrated; I have a calm about the events that is amazing. I believe I'm so overwhelmed with the love around me and so secure in what we are attempting to do. The only thing that haunts me is whether I should take another series of chemo for our trip west. I would then have to be retested out there to determine the formula again... or shall I give up on chemo?

Yesterday I spent all morning at the hospital for tests and drawing liquid from my chest again. Thank God for Esther; it was not easy. Don picked me up at the hospital and we took a drive. Nurse Mary came in the afternoon. I truly see my life slowing down and I cry at the slightest provocation. I've not been able to work, or play my instruments. Today I feel like an invalid. My left chest area hurts and I hate to use my last pain pills till I get some more. I think Don is losing it. Today I got a call from the electric company saying Don didn't sign his name on the check, and then later a call from the hardware store saying Don left something there on the counter. It reminds me of the time years back when Don had just gone to the store to get a frozen turkey. When he was returning home he thought he'd make a quick stop at the library to renew a book. Inadvertently he carried the turkey into the library in one hand, the book in the other. Maggie, the librarian, has never let us forget it.

We will be glad when things get back to normal. I wonder what normal will be.

"Those we hold most dear never truly leave us;
They live on in the kindnesses they showed,
The comfort they shared, and the love
They brought into our lives."

- *Unknown*

We still love to cuddle in bed; then all troubles and fears fade away as we whisper our love to each other. No, we won't be able to grow old together. Well my weepy week is over and I feel strong again; isn't it weird? Maybe this journal will show you how unstable life is with cancer.

We picked up our beautiful Bounder RV today, and then stopped to have dinner. I sat there and cried, poor Don. He tried so hard to make me feel good, but I have no appetite and even feel a little nervous when I eat lately. I can't stand the thought that my joy of eating is now being taken away. The doctor thinks my reactions are a result of the pain medication.

The RV purchase came about in a very strange way. The new ones all seemed to be way out of our budget, but there were a couple used ones in Crystal Lake that looked attractive. Then I noticed one in the paper that was advertised for $22,000, which included a small Chevette car. The owner said he had just driven it to an RV lot this week, but that he could possibly convince the proprietor to allow him to sell it. We made plans to visit him the following week. The next day our friends, Jim Rossiter and his wife, stopped to see us and brought a beautiful sheep's wool chair covering. Jim was once a guitar student, but we hadn't seen him for two years. We sat talking and I told him of our interest in buying an RV. He said he thinks a friend of his wants to sell one. Jim said he knows the RV is a gem because they had borrowed it for a trip at one time. "Give me the phone. I'll call him right now." Jim talked to the owner about our interest and he put him on the phone with me. You guessed it; it was the same man I had just spoken with and had made arrangements with for the following week. I'll bore you no longer. We bought it.

Now there's a new wrinkle...constipation! Since my doctor is so hard to reach, I'll call Esther. Don became irritated that he can never contact Dr. Ritzman, so he vented his frustration with her secretary; I hope it did some good.

Good news! We found the ideal couple to rent our first floor. These are friends who have been coming to the Singalong, he more than she, and love it. They are David and Judy Ashby. Dave has a treasure of nice guitars and feels the music room will be his paradise. Judy is an equestrian, but she likes the idea of being a kind of hostess at the Singalongs. When Dave talked to me at first about renting, I thought he seemed so quiet and sad, so I told him. Ben Rosenfield told us that Dave and Judy would be excellent. So we had a meeting with them and loved their attitude. They will move on the first of November which is when we will vacate to our 'nest.'

Just got a call from a friend asking for a copy of ten of my favorite recipes...why not? The real irony of me passing out recipes is that I seldom use one because I'm usually concocting something "with a little this and a little that." For instance, bread baking always seems a big deal to people. I can show you how to do it in ten minutes on video.

Now I'm getting to the end of this journal, so I'll have to start a new one. I want you kids to know this is my last love act for you, don't forget! Laugh often and much. Win the respect of intelligent people and the affection of children, knowing that even life had breathed easier because you had lived. I don't know where I read that; it's not original.

One more thing I need to say to you. I feel our problems we have with alcohol in our family is really a family problem, and it troubles me when you think you don't have a problem. If you really love others, don't invite the occasion to indulge. I love you.

One of my desires was to record some favorite songs with Don so we could give our children a sample of our kind of music. Then in October we thought why not make it available to our Singalong audience. My breathing was deteriorating so rapidly that we almost gave up on recording but for the encouragement of our friend, Mike Moutrie, who said he had a studio at his house with all the latest equipment, and it would cost us very little. It came at a time when we were getting ready to move. We scheduled a Sunday in November just prior to our departure for California. We knew it would not be the quality we could hope for, but we got a commitment from Mike O'Regan and Karen to help us out, narrowed our list to thirty songs, and drove to Buffalo Grove for the six-hour stint. We knew also we would have no time for retakes. By the end of the day my breathing was nil, but my curiosity was satisfied. We had a tape.

November 1993. Where was I? I must summarize the last two weeks because they are crucial. I've left my dear Woodstock for the last time, I'm sure, and each detail seems now so monumental to me that it's hard to know which is more important. If you can imagine leaving your friends, your home for the last time, to die...does that speak to you?

I noticed Eunice walking alone around our property the morning of our departure, and I knew it had to be. She was closing the book. The little guest houses she so beautifully decorated, the garden where she labored in prior years, pulling each weed. She loved the beauty in things that others abhorred: an ordinary thistle, the yard full of dandelions, the ground cover of leaves in the fall, the scrawny berry tree in the backyard she insisted on keeping so the birds could feed. I saw her take a seat on one of the stumps from the maple tree I had cut down...I know her prayer was to live, but her beautiful body was devastated.

The Ashbys seemed as elated to live in our house as we were to have them. Becky was the right fixture for life in the basement and the continuation of bread-making; she and we couldn't have been more pleased. She was so easy to get along with, and in her quiet way got the job done.

Our garage apartment, "the nest," was finished, thanks to nephew Dan, and it was all ready for Don when he returns. I stood in the room, alone, one more time, saw the beautiful bed where Don and I had held each other through tears, looked at our picture hanging on the wall, taken years ago before I knew...two lovers. The family picture of those I had birthed and the love I have for them. Sure, I cried, because I wanted to stay, but the time was right to go. "Good-bye things, good-bye friends. I'm headed for the River Jordan."

Eunice had made her decision several days ago about not continuing chemo. Caremark Nurse Mary was here one more time; I left them alone. She would take no more chemo and when she arrives in California she will immediately visit Dr. Paroly who will have her records and will have recommendations to make for her.

The November all-day Singalong was just as spectacular as it was billed. The Francois appeared to carry the bulk of the load, but they wanted it that way. For twelve hours there was continuous sound by well-known folk musicians from the Chicago area who each donated half-hour stints. The audience was continually changing during the day. Some people no doubt stayed for it all, and me, I sat in the audience most of the evening and alternated between crying and laughing and hugging. Heaven seemed so near...or was this it? I couldn't tell!

I must back up. We wanted to leave for California the next day, but two events were scheduled that we couldn't miss. Val Gitlin, the creative arts director at the Woodstock Opera House had told me that Maya Angelou was going to be here in November. She knew I would want to be present. Two years prior she and I were discussing her book club and she told me they were each going to suggest a book title. "Oh you should all read the new book by Maya Angelou," I said. "In fact, why don't you schedule her for the Opera House?" Val hadn't heard of Angelou so I gave her my book to read. Val was delighted with the book and subsequently had Angelou's commitment to come to the Opera House in November, so I didn't want to leave for California until after her appearance.

Also, the friends at Reba Place in Evanston where we were once members, had asked if Don and I would share an evening of our music with them. We certainly wanted to do that before we left, but the only date was the middle of November. The date with Reba Place happened on a Friday night and we left the next morning for California. Our evening at Reba Place included hours of reminiscing over the past twenty years since we've been gone. There was more crying over my prognosis, and a lot of joy in singing together.

Another event which tied in with the Reba Place visit must be mentioned. Earlier Eunice alluded to a telephone conversation she had with her father in September. I was present during that conversation. I saw an expression of pain on Eunice's face, so I hurried to an extension phone. Her father was gently rebuking Eunice for what he thought were ungodly ways, specifically not going to church, and singing folk songs instead of Christian songs. I was losing it, and was afraid of upsetting Pop if I would get on the phone. Instead I watched as Eunice, with tears in her eyes, was explaining with the little breath she had that God was real to her. She spoke of the spiritual development in her life and the practical ways this was being demonstrated. She reminded him of the "Peace Award" given to us several years before. Pop quoted Bible verses, and said, "Remember the Devil comes like an angel of light." Eunice did not let him off easy, but soon wearied of these futile religious arguments that have separated good people over the centuries; however, this stayed heavy with her till her last breath in January.

When our friend Father Brown from Reba Place heard of this encounter, he immediately wrote a letter to Pop although they had never met. He sent a copy to us; it was a letter of love, pleading for understanding and a better grip of a larger God than Pop was allowing. For that reason, also, we wanted to visit with Father Brown and express our appreciation.

Likewise our friends Esther and John Hackman wrote to Pop in a similar vein, as well as Eunice's brother-in-law Conrad Wetzel. Eunice felt satisfied in knowing that others helped to resolve an issue that struck at her heart. She had little energy to wrestle with a problem so profound, so was content to quiet herself and listen to the Spirit.

November 22, Monday: The next morning, four days before Thanksgiving 1993, we waved "Good-bye" to those who had gathered in our driveway and I gave one last look at the place of my dreams. Our first stop was just outside of Woodstock at the Farm and Fleet store parking lot where John and Esther had arranged to meet us for a send-off breakfast in our RV. The Hackmans are our closest friends and it was a tough tearing away. Esther had been my most trusted nurse through all the frustrating two and a half years of my illness and we talked and prayed and cried so often together. The four of us sat there for one hour trying to make sense of it all, but then we finally gave our farewells and drove south towards St. Louis—Tulsa—Albuquerque—Phoenix—San Diego.

> "They say you learn the most
> From your most difficult experiences.
> What a stupid system!" - *Unknown*

Last night, the second night of our trip, was rough. I was glad my teacher, Esther, told me to take Adavan if I would get a panic attack. I sensed it was coming, so I didn't allow it to develop too far. Night time can be scary far away from home with the wind blowing a fierce gale across the highway. There were loud highway noises, big trucks, and a new pain developing in my shoulder...what is it?

During the day it wasn't too bad; our candlelit breakfasts and our crying sessions three or four times a day were mixed with a few hands of cards and lots of music. Thanks to Hackmans and Francois' we were given a beautiful boom box with CD and the works. What a gift of love. It's now 6:00 a.m. We decided to get up early this morning, since Don couldn't sleep, so we pulled out of the KOA campground in northern Texas and headed west.

Breakfast and health routines are over and we settle in. Don is obliging me by traveling 50 or 55 mph. So glad it's not windy today with all the trucks and cars whizzing by. What a beautiful rig we have, so much space, and comfortable. Thanks to all of you who made it possible.

We're now in New Mexico and it looks like desert. I keep wondering where the nearest hospital is located. At least Don has a telephone installed in case of emergency. We've allowed ourselves four days of driving since we would like to pull up at Dean's house for their evening Thanksgiving dinner. Colleen is the only one who knows we're coming. Our third night we pulled into a nice trailer camp outside Phoenix, just four hours from our destination.

Thursday, November 25, Thanksgiving Day: The next morning as we drove Rte. 10 across the desert towards L.A. it was so windy that Don had to stop and tie down the awning attached to the side of the RV. Our timing couldn't have been much better. We drove into Fallbrook, Dean's hometown north of San Diego, about 5:30 p.m., stopped at the Shell station to call Dean because we needed to disconnect the little Chevette from the RV in order to get up Dean's driveway. Peter came out to help us and what a reunion we had as we drove up to the house.

All the clan was there. Holly, Jill, and Colleen had the turkey and trimmings all ready. I was so proud of all of them. Hans and Sherry would be arriving during the Christmas week. We are so happy with our daughters-in-law.

We were eager to see Ken and Phee, our local musician friends who had bought their house from Dean several years before. They were on their way over to see us. With them were Diane, the nurse we had not met, and her husband Bob. The six of us sat in the RV and talked where it was much more quiet than in the house. Co brought dessert for all of us and then I gave them each some gifts I had brought along.

After Ken and Phee left I got down to business with Diane about my illness, and we agreed on some immediate steps. They both were very helpful and knew of the seriousness of my condition. They referred me to Dr. Paroly who I will see as soon as I can make an appointment. Diane is so good; she also had many conversations with Esther by phone who shared with her the medical lingo and the urgency of treatment. What a God-send! So now I have two wonderful nurses, wonderful kids, and a wonderful husband. What more could I ask for? Oh well, I guess I would have at least one more wish....

I went to bed feeling much better.

It's now Saturday. Jake is outside with his friend Kenny. Don is at the table typing a letter that might be sent to our friends back home. This RV is so great. We can each have our little corner. It's time to get up and start my ritual: eat breakfast filled with fiber.

Colleen is something to watch; she is always getting someone food or helping the kids; she has boundless energy. Tom, Co's fiancé, has been especially helpful, too. I learned his mother died of cancer. The CD music is playing in the background, the California sun is piercing through the avocado trees here at Dean's, and I am trying to make "lemonade out of lemons"....that's the familiar phrase I've preached to my kids when things aren't what you want them to be.

Next morning Co shows up with real coffee from the house. Then some neighbors came to see us followed by the kids. It was a good morning. We've made arrangements with everyone that if we don't want to be disturbed we'll put a sign on the door window; it's been working fine. Co brought us the most delicious corn soup, Caesar salad, and pineapple this evening. Kayleigh then wanted to read me a couple books while Don and Jake play. Dean is doing pretty well as a single parent to Kayleigh, seven, and Jake, six, who usually spend every other weekend with their mother Kelly, who lives in Temecula, about a twenty-minute drive. We like Kelly. The divorce does not appear to have been bitter, but what are the kids thinking? Dean received custody because Kelly was pursuing a career, and Dean's real estate brokerage was keeping him occupied with some degree of flexibility to provide for the kids.

Before evening closed, the kids wanted my "song bag" which is my music entertainment puppet bag which they adore hearing every night. Sometimes I let each of them use one of the bags to be the teacher. When the dishes were done, the others came in the room and joined us for a wonderful gathering of fun games. When the kids went to bed, we all sat around and played cards. Everyone wants to pamper me. Somewhere around midnight we went to the RV, Don fell asleep, and I wasn't finished organizing my music and playing some instruments quietly.... Good night.

Situating the RV at Dean's house was very convenient. He had even attached us to his phone system with a cable. Being near the grandkids is nice. We had looked around at RV campsites thinking we needed privacy, but what we have here is perfect, so we're staying. Tim, Holly, and Bryan, and another son Jason who lives with Darla live in San Diego, which is about an hour south of Fallbrook on Rt. 15. Jill lives with her three children, also a single parent, about fifteen minutes from Tim; and Peter lives another fifteen minutes from Jill, so the clan is within shouting distance. Colleen is a cook on a tanker or freighter, cooking for twenty to twenty-five hungry men. She works three or four months on, then one or two months off.

I'm looking at the lovely wall quilt hanging in the RV bedroom; it came from Esther. It adds the neatest bit of hominess. The vent in the ceiling allows me to see the beautiful blue sky and hear the birds singing; what a precious day. I'm feeling so very good even though I've had to increase my morphine level a few days ago. My back was hurting so bad. This morning my constipation was relieved so all's well with the world. I miss you....

November 29: This is Monday. Yesterday was a good day with the family at Tim's house. Nice chance to talk to Holly. The men were playing basketball. Good food that I could even enjoy. I don't like to be morbid about my death, but we find it easy to talk about it with our friends and family; I think it would make dying so difficult if you pretended life would go on forever. The kids are trying to survive without me. We played some cards.

The night has descended and with it the coyotes are howling a mile up the canyon, then our dogs respond. It offsets the sound of Don snoring beside me...oh yes, I wanted to finish about yesterday. When everyone was within earshot, I said I wanted us to gather together for a surprise. Don had printed a two-sided sheet of songs for us to use at times like these. I wasn't sure everyone would go for it, but it was a huge success. The young kids especially love to sing together and I hope we do this more often. Each time we gather I remind myself it might be my last. After much gabbing we left for Dean's house one hour north.

This morning I'm waiting for Nurse Diane to come to talk and settle some questions. Wow...sometimes I get a mysterious neck pain that I can take care of with liquid morphine, but I am cautious about how fast I want to rely on Roxanol; we call it "Roxy." These are some new twists that Don and I try to deal with when we can't consult with Dr. Paroly or Diane. After a delicious meal made by Colleen, we sat in the RV and played cards. I'm so glad I have some distractions that I enjoy. Also I'm giving very elementary piano lessons to Tom and Co on the casio. Time for bed...and I always hope for sleep. I'll read till I'm too tired and then sleep. Don is already snoring. I love you.

Friday: I'm nervous about meeting my new Dr. Paroly. I have these spells, but then I can talk it out with Don or Co. The music routine heals me. From the accordion to the psaltry to the guitar or banjo. So we marched to the doctor armed with our artillery of papers and folders. Co and Don were with me. Immediately I heard a loudmouthed nurse call, "Eunice Mast." I was pleased at the first sight of him; kind, oldish, and down to business. I could see right away he knew the seriousness of my situation. He answered all my fifty questions and he began discussing my course of action. He said he didn't want to pressure me into anything I didn't want to do. He wants me to consider taking an oral chemo that doesn't have the serious side effects of my other chemo. I was not interested in pursuing anything that was powerful enough to give me side effects. At least if I take the pill I'm doing something that might reduce the tumors, just a twenty-five percent chance, he said. I feel assured that if it has few side effects, it is not very powerful. We should watch what happens and just treat the symptoms as they appear and enjoy life to the fullest.

I felt better. So there wasn't much good news to report; the nervousness is gone. Co and I had a good talk about things as we drove towards San Diego. We were going to meet Ken and Phee to hear a guitarist. I was so excited to listen to music again. How much I miss the Singalongs and my music room which I spent years in creating. The coffee house, Choices, was attractive and we sat down to hear Johnny Walker and Sam Hinton (Seeger types).

December 4: Saturday dawned bright and beautiful, but I was having a "downer" for no good reason. I stayed in the RV crying till Don helped me through it and I decided it was time to go in and be with the others. Peter came and we all enjoyed another good meal by Co. Peter loved reading *Freddie The Leaf*—a children's story about dying that I wanted to read to Kayleigh and Jake. Then all of us drove into Fallbrook and watched the two-hour parade.

When we returned, I discovered that I had not taken the cake out of the oven. So being resourceful, I cut off the burnt edges, squeezed on plenty of frosting, dressed it up with roses and it looked pretty nice. Don's birthday cake was for such a great man, and he didn't flinch a bit about its burnt taste. Here it is the first week of December and I am still living.

...and the mail today had just what I needed. A letter from a Sherry Brown. I don't know her well, but she comes to the Singalong. Her letter was the lift that gave me additional assurance of the "stuff of life"....

Dear Don and Eunice,
I had my first child the summer of the Woodstock (NY) Folk Festival, and part of me always wished that I could have been there. I would have enjoyed the performers and perhaps felt the freedom that I've heard existed. I was just a teenager when Martin marched on Washington and the Chicago 7 rioted to protest and create a change. I always wished I had been more vocal and helped to make that change. But in my own way I will be able to reminisce in years to come about something that had much less notoriety, yet such wonderful subdued impact. I can say, "Yes, I was at the Masthouse monthly singalong more than once." I would like to let you know from just one more person how much it meant to those of us who shared your home once a month. I'll never forget the first time I came wondering what I was in for. I couldn't believe anyone would just leave their doors open for those who choose to enter and share in the singing. Didn't your mothers teach you to be afraid of strangers? And so instead you made me feel that just maybe in a world where my newspaper is full of negatives and war and hatred that there is still good and people really could be trusted.

I couldn't believe that you had decorated with red flocked wall paper and gold cherubs and macrame and an umbrella table. Or that your lower level had booths with good old checkers and chess games asking to be played. I never had seen such abandoned disregard for "normalcy" and symmetric decorating techniques, but instead I saw that it welcomed and worked and excited every sense and I couldn't wait to look and see something different somewhere else or how "boring" my home was by comparison, and I promised myself to dare to be more adventuresome. I couldn't believe the talent that I got to see. I'll never forget the evening an older man that in my judgmental way looked like he had retired from a factory line came to the microphone to sing with a voice that made me gasp because of its beauty. Young and old were brought together to share through the love of music and the generation gap disappeared.

But I think the best thing I got out of the evenings was sharing the experience with not only my husband but our seventeen-year old son who returned, bringing his friends more than once. He looks at the world with fresher more hopeful eyes. And as he goes on he will also be able to say he was at the Masts when he was a kid. All those wonderful evenings full of experiences, sights, and sounds most definitely will affect him too. I feel I would be remiss in not saying "Thank you" for touching so many of our lives and truly making a difference in this world. I'm so glad I had opportunity to be touched by you and yours and I wish you peace and love.   - Sherry Brown

The next morning everyone else went out to eat breakfast, but I preferred to stay home by myself to cry. Sometimes the whole weight just descends on me at once. The memories of all those years of fun and music. I grabbed my guitar and started playing and singing amidst my tears till I got it all out. Don came home and we sang some more. It put me in a good mood for a candlelit dinner and cards. Then we all sat around and Don showed everyone our slides on our third Russian trip, the one where we lived with Nikitins in Moscow for two weeks, traveled with them to dachas of friends outside Moscow and to villages very few foreigners get to see. Of course, the highlight of that trip was the folk festival in Samara, where we sang before 60,000 people seated on a mountainside. The Festival was in its eighth year and was organized to honor the death of a man who had died in a swimming accident in trying to save two boys. People arrive by train, usually, from all parts of Russia, even as far away as Vladivostock. Never before have performers come from outside the Soviet Union. Samara is the new post-Soviet name for the town formerly known as Kubishev, situated on the Volga about 100 miles east of Moscow.

The Russian trips highlighted Eunice's charisma. She mentioned our friendship with the singers, Sergei and Tanya Nikitin, whom we met first on the 1988 Volga tour. One of many memories of that trip was the first night on the ship when these 200-plus passengers (100 American, 100 Russian) were scrambling to find berths, etc. I made an announcement that there would be music in the meeting room on deck for anyone interested; bring your guitar. Nearly fifty people gathered; Eunice took it from there. She announced that since we don't know each other we'll go around the room, introduce ourselves, and sing a song or two. The Nikitins sang first, the old Josh White song that still brings tears to my eyes, "I Know Moonlight." When they invited us to live with them the summer of 1990, Eunice became the focus in any party that we attended. She bedecked Zyama Gerdt, the famous Russian dramatist, with a "BEARS" headband; she showed Sergei's mother how to bake a cake, and how to conduct a birthday party—without being able to converse in Russian proved hilarious. She endeared herself to everyone by her openness and love. The following summer she learned of cancer.

Without a doubt, Eunice's open attitude about her own impending death unmasked us all. It allowed the children to speak of their feelings more easily. To hear her say, "I'm not afraid to die," was not surprising because she was such a dynamic teacher in showing us how to live.

My son, Hans, writes....

"I will never forget the last Christmas 1993 that I spent with Mom. Although she was ill, somehow she managed to smile. We played cards in the RV, ate chocolates, and had frank discussions about life, and death.

"Before I left to return to Chicago, I met her one last time. She was lying in bed and her smile was faded. I told her that I loved her and how lucky I felt to be her son. She said I was a good son, and that she was proud of me. But, I'm proud of my mother. I will always remember the love and generosity she had for others; the simple things in life were always what gave her so much joy and satisfaction in life.

"I have so many memories...

- the many days I would awake to her piano playing outside my bedroom door;
- coming home to her singing and playing wildly on the piano, banjo, or guitar;
- the excitement she got from finding a great bargain at a garage sale—a gift for someone;
- preparing her eleven-course mels and homemade bread for visiting guests;
- and the endless games, such as blowing bubbles, limbo, dictionary, and concentration we would play together.

"The one wish she had was for all her children to be as happy in their lives as she was in hers, a hard act to follow. She has given all of us a perfect outline in which to pattern our lives. She taught me so much and she has given me more than I could ever ask for. In return, all I can hope to do is continue her legacy of generosity, love, and a zest for life. In this way, she will always be with me."

-Hans read this at Eunice's memorial on January 30, 1994.

I had trouble sleeping because of neck pains during the night. I just imagined cancer spreading to all of my bones, so I got out my bottle of Roxy and took a swig; it is very fast acting, but doesn't last as long as the morphine taken through the groshong. The night was long as I lay and listened to the dogs and coyotes ruling the canyons. Hope tomorrow is better.

Yep. The next day was better. I did a lot of practicing with Don. What a beautiful day. I made a fruit salad and set the table for my lunch guests, Diane and Phee. About 2:00 p.m., Don announced we were going to a movie, "My Life." Co and Tom and Dean went with us. The story was about a young fellow dying of cancer. We missed the first ten minutes but caught up with the plot fast. Co and Tom sat in back of us. At one point Co handed the three of us tissues. There was a lot of emotion near the end. I grabbed Dean's hand on one side and Don's on the other and we were all crying. The experience was a treasure. I feel so good about the growth of the kids in accepting and talking about death.

The phone rang early this morning. My brother John was wondering what we'd think about them bringing Pop and Mom out to see us. I knew the background of this idea was the phone conversation I had with Pop earlier in the fall. Also, I'm sure the letters regarding that phone call which he received from Conrad, Father Brown, and Hackmans must have weighed on him. He wanted to see me before I die. John was bothered about Pop's intransigence. "You have to consider the source and not be overly worked up," he said to me. Easy for him to say; put yourself in my shoes. Don't forget this is the same Pop we all grew to fear, like it or not! Now I'm not supposed to worry about what he says. Now as I reflect again on that phone call from Pop in September, I am still hurt real bad, but I also have a pity for him. I have never doubted his love for me because of his care for me, but he never told me that he loved me, rather I felt he was often critical of how I looked, or what I did. The phone call only reinforced that attitude. I hoped and prayed there would be a way to resolve this before I die.

When you're dying, every encounter can either break you down or support your own confidence. I was certainly reinforced spiritually by the voice in my soul, by Don, and by my close friends that I shared with. Now this ninety-year-old couple was flying 3,000 miles to see me before I die. To me that was a good sign because they hate to fly. I'm not at ease about seeing them. Although pleased, I don't anticipate they will ask forgiveness or show much emotion; they are accustomed to just symbolizing a feeling. Sometimes that's hard to read.

I remember one time years ago when we went to Pennsylvania to visit them, I thought I would just "take the bull by the horns" and give Pop a big hug, a most unfamiliar greeting in our family. Of course it felt artificial, but I satisfied myself that although I can't control him, I can follow my own instincts, and no one can take that away. John told me on the phone that Pop and Mom were surprised when they read the letters I referred to.

"Of course, you can come out with them," I told John. I have felt so good about my relationship with John and about his expressions of love to us and to our children. I'm proud of him. He has had to be the mediator and family counselor with my parents because all the other siblings live in other parts of the country. Don and I sat at the foot of the bed and discussed this unusual turn of events. They would be arriving in a couple weeks if they can still get tickets. John will let us know very soon. How shall we plan for them? I knew that my health would deteriorate much faster if I become anxious, so I stilled my soul and allowed God to hear me.

There was still another episode that had occurred during the fall that caused me to hurt. My sister Lois had sent me a note following her visit to the September Singalong where friends had gathered to express their love for me. She thought I should have given more glory to God. In what ways, I asked myself, does God receive glory? I tried to understand Lois; we've always been close, and I tried to talk to her about this concern, but I don't have the feeling that I was understood either.

Don and I feel so happy in the direction our lives have taken over the last forty years, that I give thanks to God always. I haven't had any more anxiety attacks for days, what a relief. I'm so happy my parents want to come; I'm sure they want to reassure me of their love...we'll see. It was such a beautiful California morning that Don and I decided to go to a few garage sales on our way to the doctor. Why do I love to still go to garage sales in my condition? It's cheaper than therapy, I've always told people. We arrived at the hospital in time for my chest x-ray; the doctor wanted to see the progression of my cancer, as if I didn't know. It is very tight in my chest and my discoloration is rampant.

After some piano lessons for Co and Tom, Nurse Diane arrived for a chat; she's a gem. She gives me the comfort I need. Another development is that I need a "rubber tire" to hold my uterus and bladder in place. Oh brother, what else is falling apart in this old chassis? Diane found a doctor that specializes in that, so she pulled a few strings and got me an appointment sooner than otherwise would have been possible. I have a few more fears that I need to tell him about. The night comes on with the usual candlelit dinner, cards, and a kiss.

Next morning it's more of the same. Now the pills seem to bring about a nausea toward food. I hate to lose that part of my life also. I had enough energy to want to go downtown San Diego with the gang and go Christmas shopping. At Horton's Plaza we scattered and each did his thing. Later, we met at the theater to see the play, "A Christmas Carol," Gospel version. I was energized again. I don't know how many more of these I'll get to see.

When Don and I cuddled again that night and shared the day's memories, hugged and kissed, and talked of the years of wanderings, I felt so loved and blessed. Don soon fell asleep and I recounted all the miracles or "coincidences" that happened in my sixty years. For instance, yesterday we were watching TV while waiting for Nurse Diane when I heard Oprah say, "This week I plan to have all of the people I would love to invite over for a coffee break. The first person will be Deepak Chopra. He'll be here in a minute." As I expected, the guest was going to expound on the same subject as Lucinda, a friend of Dean's who stopped to visit me last night. Also Colleen had just given me his book to read: *Ageless Body, Timeless Mind*. Suddenly my chest started to tighten. My spirits aren't so good, maybe a bit depressed.

"If I can stop one heart from breaking,
   I shall not live in vain;
If I can ease one life the aching, or cool one pain,
   Or help one fainting robin unto his nest again,
I shall not live in vain."   *- Emily Dickinson*

I got through the night. Now I have to look forward to my visit with the doctor to examine my uterus. I've almost lost all my pride in getting embarrassed about my worn body. Dear Diane picked me up and together we went to the doctor. He was very friendly, wearing loafers with no socks; I guess this is California. He was so kind that at one point I broke out crying when he asked me to tell my situation. He wanted to be so sure I would be without pain; he sure knows my number. That is all I talk about; I want to die without pain. Esther and all my nurses tell me that I need have no worries in this day and age.

Don helped things by reading to me tonight from the book Esther gave us on what to expect during the "last" month. It was difficult for both of us, but we held hands and cried together. More TV and another night.

Tonight Don suddenly got the urge to call our friends, the Millers in Canada. To our surprise they had just turned off the video we sent them: "There was Music," the September Singalong. What lovely memories we shared over the years with the Millers. As soon as we hung up, Vic and Marie called from Indiana. Friends are forever.

Today we got a package from Dee in Woodstock telling us the little Masthouse replicas are finished and she sent us copies for all the kids. How can I ever thank everybody for their kindnesses. Well, I did just that by writing some notes. But now I'm sleepy so I'll try to disregard the barking dogs. It won't be long before Hans and Sherry will be visiting. All the kids will be here for Christmas. Someone has planned for a family picture....won't I be a pretty sight!

So yesterday was a low; today is a high most of the day, trying not to be fearful that feelings of depression will return; it's so terrible. I truly had very little experience with these kinds of days before. We sat around tasting Co's cookies. I just watch her, knowing her energy and enthusiasm would be fun to have again, but also knowing it won't be. Still I can see myself in her, and that is joy; maybe that's why we named her Colleen Joy. How I used to enjoy cleaning the house, cooking for whomever stops in, practicing whenever I get a chance, running with Don to garage sales, and on and on. I watched her work with a bunch of kids who were helping her cook. She said she felt like Julia Childs. I went with Don to town to recharge the RV and I was impressed again with the beauty of Fallbrook and of Dean's acre of avocado trees lining the driveway.

Tonight it was nice by the fireplace in Dean's living room. Don had tucked Jake in bed and then we all sat around talking. Pete sat next to me and we held hands and I felt so good about him. He opened up to me in such a wonderful way, telling me how nice it was to have parents like us and for all the values we taught him. He wants the same values. I treasured that night. We discussed some plans for the upcoming visit of my folks, maybe some discussions and some readings on the subject of death. I'm glad I'm not anxious about the visit. The kids want to do hymn singing with them and some carol singing. I'll have to get out my folders of songs we copied.

I must admit a little nervousness if they expect to involve us in a theological discussion. This is not the time and place to discuss what Jesus taught. I don't want to hurt them, but I feel secure in my understanding of "The Way."

Have they made God too small? Perhaps they are not excited about our "folk singing" because they misunderstand the term. In their own hymnal, they will find quite a few: "Amazing Grace," "Blessed Assurance," "Dwelling in Beulah Land," "Just a Closer Walk," "Precious Lord," "Shall we Gather at the River"; they're all there, and a thousand more that we sing regularly. Why do I bother with these trifles; I guess because I love and care! They feel our peace songs are too humanistic. I guess that's because we are humans! Lord, give us wisdom and hearts full of love and light from above. Thank you, God, for your love and peace and joy in the midst of this body of cancer. To bed.

Don is already sleeping; that's my time to write when I'm alone. The dogs are barking and all is well with the world. Dean just got home from a date with Lucinda. I can't wait to meet her again.

At 1:00 a.m., I got awake with this recurring neck pain; the bottle of Roxanol is real handy for a fast-acting cure, thanks to Esther's advice. I was just dreaming that I got company and it was Jackie Kauffman. I like her. It seems we're on the same "page." I was so upset because I noticed the outside door to a cellar room was open and it must have been open when we were driving and what fell out, I wonder. The whole dream was about my compartment full of kids' show stuff. When will I erase my feverish activity with creating shows, bubbles, puppets? I can remember I was developing puppet shows before "Sesame Street" was on the drawing board, back in the early 1960's.

Friday, December 10: A letter today from a Woodstock friend who brought her sons faithfully to my kids' shows once a month.

"...on Wednesday Colin, my six-year-old, started to sing, 'May there always be sunshine, may there always be blue skies,' then he stopped and said, 'That was Eunice's song. They are learning it at school in French and Spanish. I asked my music teacher if we could dedicate it to Eunice, and she said "Yes."'
Thank you for all the gifts, you have given so many."
- *Lisa Roberts*

A strange thing happened to me today. I walked into a bookstore near home and hunted for a good interesting book to read at night. I kept coming back to *Love Can Build a Bridge* by Naomi Judd, who had to give up her career because of cancer.

Finally, I bought it even though it cost $15.00. She found such an inner strength to heal herself. Later, when we were getting ready for bed, Don called me to come watch TV. He said a country singer was going to be interviewed. He didn't know I had just bought her book. Is that a coincidence or what? In the front of her book is a quote by Abe Lincoln that says: "The written word may be man's greatest invention. It allows us to converse with the dead, the absent, and the unborn!" Judd also starts out with an interesting thought about listening to the light within you, sitting perfectly still. I wonder if she heard of the Quakers.

Next morning...I told Peter to come out to the RV this morning about 8:00 a.m. I wanted to make him breakfast before he had to leave to begin work building decks. We sat with candles, shredded wheat, juice, and donuts. We watched a video show of some of the Singalong concerts. He liked "Dos Boys." Then gradually the other family members who were at Dean's came out and joined us. I'm so happy they enjoy our Singalong activities; I know it's not quite their style of music, but they are impressed by the spirit of our gatherings at Masthouse; it's a love community and love is God.

I'm going back to sleep.

I woke up with that shoulder pain so I went for more "Roxy." Nurse Diane said you never need to be afraid of taking too much. I stayed in bed, read, and visited with whomever showed up. Had a long talk with Colleen over coffee and cookies. Who cares about getting fat now!

That's the second nice thing about having cancer I've heard: "You don't need to worry about getting fat" or "You don't need to worry about getting cancer anymore." Don is peeling eight pounds of apples now so I can make apple dumplings for tonight. I just got the mail today with a letter about the December Singalong, the first one without us in command. Steve and Sylvia are just naturals for the job and they do it with such dedication. Thanks, guys. The report is that some people don't want to attend because we aren't there. Now isn't that a little silly. I think they're trying to make me feel good. You would make me feel better by coming to show support to the great group who is running it now. This is the end of a nice day, filled with games, eating, cooking, piano teaching, reading, cards. Isn't it remarkable how the days can fluctuate so much for me.

I stayed up late to read and continue my organizing kids games, etc. "Love can build a bridge" and oh do we need a lot of bridge-building.

Jill had me in stitches when she told me about her interview for a job when they asked her to describe her mother. By her description of me, the ladies thought my name must be Mary. She is taking my illness so hard. We got home from a drive and found Co cuddled up in our RV writing a letter to us. Then to bed to read this high-powered mail and a book from Esther, *Final Gifts.*

Don and I prayed for light and strength tonight. I went through another hour or so of panic and depression that comes without warning. I'm sure it must be the meds, because I don't remember ever getting depressed in my life. I'm going to take Adavan at the first sign next time.

"I can face anything except the future and certain parts of the past and present"...or "I try to take one day at a time, but sometimes several days attack me at once"...or "Right now I'm working on a fascinating project, staying alive."

Today Don and I gave Jake some special attention. Some of the time I was alone with Jake, read to him *Freddie the Leaf,* and then he helped me do some cooking. Tonight I'll play with them in the "trick bag" which they love; they can go for over two hours literally. Another good children's book about death is *Life Times.* Jake loved talking about being in the ground and then daisies growing up later on and how old you are when you die. I had heard him talking outside the RV earlier in the day with his friend, Kenny, who asked Jake, "Would you want worms to be eating your body in the ground? I wouldn't." I'm imagining his parents were discussing my death with him. Oh to be like kids!

Friday, December 17: Next day, a shift in plans. John just called saying they weren't flying out to see us till January 7-9 because of needing the fourteen-day waiting period for the cheaper tickets. I hope I'm living that long. I'll just program myself to live. So we went to San Diego today. We went to our favorite spot, Seaport Village, then to Tim's for a ham dinner made by Holly and Co. We're amazed at how I'm hanging on, although my strength is ebbing. I've pretty well decided not to go through the lung aspiration again. How much am I jeopardizing my life if I don't drain the fluid, and does it really matter if I am able to live two weeks longer and not go through the pain. As long as I have my bottle of "Roxy," it doesn't matter.

I only took one swig in twenty-four hours, but then I get the longer-acting morphine at night and sleep well. This morning I got awake at 6:00 a.m. and started reading, then sleeping and alternating like that untill Don got me breakfast in bed.

Dean, Co, and Tom came to the RV and talked to us about the future. These are rich family times I've often dreamed about. I'm so happy they can air their feelings about death; that's music to my ears! Then in the middle of the conversation we got a phone call from Taj Mahal in Hawaii. He had visited our home in Woodstock several years ago and we had kept contact. Don had called him about the trip to Russia, and he was explaining his busy schedule made it impossible. That phone connection to my bed is such a blessing; thank you, Dean.

Don and I bought a piano for Dean from the "Want-ads" today. The owner said her friend just died of breast cancer and was reluctant to talk to her own family about it. How sad! Now I can pound on a piano again. That joy I learned from Mom. Rarely do I spend much time thinking of all the instruments in my home in Woodstock and the fun I had going from one to the other. I suppose there's no remorse because there was not much choice for me. Don and I have come through some very big and important decisions together these last few months: the prospect of dying, selling our treasures, moving from the house into an RV, and leaving our friends in Woodstock for the last time!

Colleen spent some time talking about her joy of giving up alcohol. She attends one or two AA meetings a day. She says they are spiritually fulfilling as well as instrumental if she wants to stay clean. There's so much support and understanding of the aspects of the disease and she's learning how to break the vicious cycle.

Tonight again I notice a big difference in my breathing ability and am convinced that I don't have much longer. I told Don not to feel bad if I die soon and fast. I'm not going to get pumped out every week in order to live a little longer. God, I hope it won't be a prolonged death, that's all I ask. I already feel so grateful for answers to my other requests of feeling at peace with my soul and with God and family, and the richness of life, even now.

Slept good. Got awake at 7:00 a.m. Don read more of Kubler-Ross to me. When we read I get the feeling I'm in the last stage, which is acceptance, and yet I have hope. Actually, I have been in the acceptance stage for five or six months, but have tried to go on with my fun life. Bill and Marina just called. It's so nice to talk to people back home. They haven't forgotten me.

Now Don is tuning the instruments for me to practice a bit. I still have some breath left for that.

Just had a wonderful lunch with Phee. She is also taking Tamoxifin for an initial stage of breast cancer. Her story is a little scary. One year ago when she learned I had cancer she became paranoid about her own condition so she went to the doctor about her lumps. When the doctor seemed to try to make her relax and not worry about it, she became incensed and ordered him to take a biopsy. He did and it turned out positive. Life for women is scary. How do you know what to do? I cherish my time with her because we get right down to the point. She wants so badly to be available for me in these last months. She just went through two other friends' cancer deaths. Can you imagine? Another evening of games and fun.

Next morning we had another good chat with Dean. He came out to the RV in his housecoat and told us of his thoughts of the book by Wayne Dwyer. To watch our kids mature physically was rewarding, but then to see them grow spiritually and be willing to ask questions and share thoughts about the future and about this life is even more blessed. Time for food preparation for tonight: acorn squash stuffed with maple syrup, sausage, red cabbage, and a baked cauliflower, taboli salad, apple crisp with ice cream. If I keep busy with what I love to do I won't think of my own condition nearly as much.

We were ready; the guests came. Co served in her elegant style just like I often dreamed she would do and Tom is a wonderful partner. Just then the phone rang...Eunice, for you. It was Jackie Kaufman. Everyone who had gathered at her home for Christmas fun and food wanted to say, "Hi." Do we feel loved or what? Then we had a hymn sing which was something our friends were unaccustomed to. Everyone loved it and wanted more. Even our own children had not had much training with harmony singing even though some are accomplished guitarists.

Sunday, December 19: By midnight everyone had gone home. The weight of the day was heavy; and I knew I had overworked. That caused me to cry uncontrollably with Don holding me like a baby. I called Dr. Paroly the next day and had to tell him through my tears that I had trouble breathing. He was very kind and explained some options. If possible I should make an effort at relaxing and breathing more slowly. He explained that I could have an oxygen tank in the RV to use whenever the need arises.

Diane came over the next day and we discussed these options. She is able to get the tank for me. We also will want to be connected with Hospice soon. Their care is necessary when we feel that I will need to be staying in the RV most of the time. Then I got a wonderful letter from my dear Esther. It made me want to call her immediately. It helps me so much to have trusted people like this around to help me make decisions. Think of all the cancer people that need to rely on Hospice or someone to help them through. God, help us.

We got some nice mail. Letter and book from Vic and Marie *When I'm Alone, Thoughts of Prayer and Comfort.* Don often comes up to me and kisses me and asks, "Shall we pray?" He is absolutely the best in helping me through these days. I could have the moon!

Co is sick today so I don't want to be near her. That's disappointing because she is such a gem. I want to see Jill more often, too, but she lives an hour away and with such a busy schedule she can only phone occasionally.

Peter is here again and brought a stool near my bed. We had a nice chat. I asked him if he had anything he needed to talk about before I die, but he really didn't. He just wanted to be near me as much as he could. So we just talked about how good things were going for him right now and how he was making some changes in his life.

Don read more of Kubler-Ross to me tonight. It's helpful to hear how other people handle these situations when faced with death. Maybe this journal will even help someone cope with cancer. We're not giving up hope. God, please heal me. Peace is not the absence of conflict, but the ability to deal with it. Thank you, God, for a warm peace feeling today. "I will lift up my eyes unto the hills. My help cometh from the Lord. Thou wilt keep him in perfect peace whose mind is stayed on thee."

I finished my Judd book last night. She gave me a lot of strength and hope. I crave to have some of her wisdom and insights. She went through much worse stuff than I did and chose to listen to her inner light and got rid of chemo. She's in remission right now. Don and I are finding more and more comfort in just centering on God.

Peter just brought me breakfast from the house. The menu was bacon, eggs, toast, juice, and coffee, and two Hershey kisses. I guess Don was cook this morning. Peter and I ate and talked. Don and I went for a cruise in the RV today. This thirty-two-foot home is so nice; I want all of you to know who helped us buy it. I read most of today because I have such little breath to walk around like I used to do. How I used to enjoy just walking from one store to the next.

More reading in *Final Gifts* tonight. We talked about dying and our feelings. The next day around noon I got a call from Ella Jenkins, Chicago. Our friendship goes back to about 1965 or 1966 when we were at Reba Place, Evanston.

This little anecdote shows again what I mean about Eunice's charisma. She and a friend walked to the nearby elementary school where Ella was performing. After the show, Eunice went up to Ella and expressed her appreciation for the program and ideas she was going to use with kids' programs.

"Would you come home and have lunch with us?" Eunice asked.

"Of course, I would," Ella said. Eunice dashed home and concocted some delicacy out of her welfare budget that was "heavenly." Before Ella left she had bought a Martin baritone uke that Eunice's friend Joan owned. Many years later when we lived in Woodstock, Ella was appearing at the Opera House for a concert which Eunice attended. When Ella spotted her in

the audience, she insisted Eunice come up on the stage and sing with her. Following the concert Ella came home to eat with us and Eunice had prepared a delicious pizza which Ella was drooling over. When Eunice was ready to serve her on the deck, she asked Ella if she'd like large, medium, or small. Without much hesitation, Ella said she wanted a small one. Hanging from a beam in the kitchen were pans of all sizes from the black frying pans measuring 12 inches in diameter to the very tiniest one, two inches across which is the one she used in serving Ella, who still refers to this little episode in her life.

Monday, December 20: I called Diane this morning and cried, telling her I needed to talk to her tonight. During the day Don and I went alone to the Oceanside beach ten miles away. We stopped on the way at a bookstore and picked up Peck's *Further Along the Road Less Traveled.* It's fun to read a book and pass it on to the kids. Already I've given them, among others, *Wouldn't Take Nothing For My Journey* and *Gather Together In My Name* by Angelou. I guess I've given my last children's show, because I just don't have the energy anymore.

Diane came tonight and we had a wonderful chat. She told me exactly what to tell and ask the doctor. She thinks I shouldn't be part of Hospice yet. She will take care of me whenever I need her. If the doctor orders my oxygen, the insurance company will take care of it. Then she checked my groshong and changed the cap which was usually my job. She made me feel good. She praised me for taking such good control of my problems, pain, constipation, etc. Phee called today when she learned I was in tears.

After another candlelit dinner, I went wild on the piano, Don sang, and Peter started reading my first diary where I bared my soul. The night enveloped me after some reading, cards, and my trusty "Roxy."

We got a load of mail today. It's so much fun to hear from our friends. Tonight Don read about one cancer patient who died in her sleep. Please, Lord, that's the way I want to go. I'm ready now. I've had a charmed life and still do, but we all gotta go sooner or later.

I just ran to the house to talk to Co and I learned that I can't do that anymore. The nurse has made an appointment with me at the hospital to be tested to see whether my blood indicates I would be eligible for insurance to cover my oxygen. Co is so worried that she's accepting my death too easily. She thinks she must be uncaring or unfeeling, or that maybe she hasn't accepted it yet. Perhaps we're talking so freely about it, it has become such a natural part of us.

Two years later, Co still has the same feelings of acceptance over Eunice's "passing over into the spiritual realm." The impact of losing such a strong force in her life gave way to a more complete understanding of the everlasting and more incredible part of us all—our eternal spirits.

I'm just exceedingly grateful that I haven't had a panic attack for a long time. I can handle anything else, it seems. Beautiful day. Actually it's the first day for a long time that I didn't take "Roxy." Don picked fifteen lemons from Dean's tree so I could make lemon pie tonight.

We are spoiled with all this fruit growing right out in the yard: avocado, lemon, grapefruit, orange, tangerine. I like to keep my hand in a little work even though I know a couple pies is about all I can manage today. I'm just happy to have enough energy to do that. Don is a great help with anything I want done.

Wednesday, December 22: Today at the hospital they took blood from the artery instead of the vein in order to tell how much oxygen is in the blood. Since it was within normal bounds, the insurance company will not compensate for an oxygen tank. We would get it anyway if it is absolutely necessary. The doctor has instructed me how to breathe so that I don't have to rely on a tank yet. Also the Hospice will get us the oxygen equipment if we want to be part of that program. We'll take it one day at a time; it's nice to have these options.

Colleen is back in circulation again. We had another delicious meal. I'm glad that food looks good again. I enjoyed some cards and our cozy RV bed with some more chapters in *Final Gifts*. Am I really going to die? What does that mean? I can hardly think of anything else when I'm alone at night. I wish I would have the energy to keep Kayleigh on a practice routine with the piano. Good night to another nice day.

I am still finding notes left by Eunice in jars, desk drawers, etc. Today I found this hastily scribbled note:
"Love is like a game of catch, the easy back and forth of an unscored ball...no points counted, no cups or medals won. Love returned with love is quite enough to keep the game going."
- Margaret Tsuda

Wednesday, December 29: Bad news. I lost this journal for about a week it seems and I haven't kept up with all the happenings. I'll summarize. Christmas day was unusual to say the least. I prepared myself emotionally and spiritually for a tough day and invited as much help from the family and friends who were available. I had volunteered to travel to the local nursing home to sing and play some carols. I knew this was my last gig so I wanted to make it the best. There were quite a few people in various degrees of alertness, but that didn't matter to me. I was doing it for me as much as for them...my last performance with my instruments. We had a wild time. It must have been a funny sight with me prancing around the room, accordion strapped tightly against all that cancer, trying to sing and breathe. I had a choice.

I was really puffing and noticed one of the ladies breathing gently from an oxygen tank. I felt like stopping and taking a drag. The hour went faster than expected and I headed straight for the van and stretched out while the others loaded the equipment. That afternoon we all gathered at Tim's for singing, gifts, and picture-taking. I was just wishing I had the energy like I used to have. The RV bed never felt better.

The next morning my chest was so constricted. If I cried, there was even more pressure and less air to breathe. We called Diane immediately and she got the Hospice ball rolling. It wasn't long before we were all set up with Hospice. They brought the tank and showed us how to work it. We can use it as little or as much as we want. It relieves the panic a bit at least. I'm ready to die now.

It's so frightening when you think you just can't breathe, even with the oxygen tube. I have to learn that skill, or panic could still set in. Hans and Sherry were here over the holidays. We had a great time.

Don and I are so impressed with the quality of the Hospice workers. What a Godsend for people who are dying and are afraid to face it. One of the nurses wanted us to tell her about ourselves. Well, she suddenly burst into tears when she saw the video of the Singalong, the love and sharing of so many wonderful people.

Food is now totally distasteful to me. I told the nurses that I don't want to be pumped out anymore. I will now just try to be comfortable. They were supportive, so I had donuts and candy for lunch to celebrate my decision. Don forgot and asked me if I wanted a hamburger that he was making. At last I got through to Don that he should not force food to keep me alive and the nurse confirmed by showing us an article that explains how the body works when food is not needed anymore. Full-time oxygen, no more food. It's enough to make me curl up and die.

Thursday, December 30: Then we got the mail, and that brought me love messages again. I've got to share one:

"Eunice, whatever lies ahead for you, please know that your life journey has been and continues daily to be an inspiration to all you have met along your way. I take comfort in knowing that whenever we meet again...for we will meet again...I will once again delight in your sparkling eyes, bright smile, warm hug, and loving words. And once again I will do my best to sing in tune, clap in time, and dance in step to your everlasting music!"
- Sue Bernstein

Becky just sent me her diary today. I wish so much we could have time to talk 'cause I could help her find a spiritual peace, and that doesn't mean you have to be going to church either or reading the Bible and praying if you don't want to. Just open yourself to the light and follow it. "Love will guide you." "Give yourself to love." My pills must be working. I don't feel like doing anything but playing cards, so that's what we're going to do, oxygen and all. I'm going to sleep now midst the howling of coyotes and the echo of the dogs.

My new Hospice nurse came today and I like her. She'll do just fine listening to my blubberings and fears and all I told her that I'm not interested in prolonging this poor quality of life. I work for each breath I take. If I take enough "Roxy" then I can breathe; but I can't think, what a tradeoff! I've enjoyed talking to lots of people on the phone. The mail is so fantastic! Don is so wonderful in showing his love and care. He tries his best to sneak food down me to keep me alive longer, but I've made up my stubborn mind that "I wanna go home...yes, I'm ready to go home to heaven to the light...to the love...to my God...to hear sweet Jordan roll...swing low, sweet chariot, come and carry me home."

Friday, December 31: It's still work to write in this journal, but it's my last testament. Probably I've repeated myself, but does it matter? Don and I quote the Twenty-third Psalm every morning for comfort. We usually end in tears, but still it is soothing. We often pray short prayers where Don is asking for me to have peace in my last days, and I interrupt by saying, "But I have peace; I don't need any more of that." We still joke around. Colleen stopped in for awhile today. We had such a wonderful talk. She has a way of comforting me that is so good. When I think how far she and I have come in our relationship in one year. We both laugh and thank God in the same breath.

Don just gave me some "Roxy" for pain in my stomach area. We've just called the doctor because I have a new worry. I'm hemorrhaging and my nurse looked concerned. She said, "That's a new one for me." That's comforting to know! It's amazing how often I've heard some nurse say that about me during my illness. I've not had a normal pattern of breast cancer at all. Esther and Joyce just called. What neat friends I have. More cards tonight. Don just built me a new nest on my bed so that I can have my upper part raised on a wedge provided by Hospice. I feel so special. More calls from home. I talked to Phyllis and Letty, our dear, dear neighbor in Woodstock. It all ended as night came on and Don kissed me good night.

We tease a lot. "I don't think you fed me lunch today. You must want me to die fast." We prayed and read some more and I noticed Don could hardly keep his eyes open.

Oh, I don't want to let go of Don tonight. I'm praying to fall asleep permanently tonight; I hope Don understands. The "Roxy" is kicking in because I fall asleep between the words I wrote. Some strange things are happening to me.
    Don is scurrying around here taking care of me so well. He thinks he would be a good nurse. Then I hear beautiful organ music. I told Don, "I think they're comin' to carry me home...I mean it! I hear it clearly." I really did want to see Pop and Mom this weekend, but that's O.K. Don would get an extra $13,000 from insurance money if I live till February 10, but I told him not to feel bad if I sneak out early.

    Monday, January 3: I had such a good sleep last night. I thank God for that. It means so much to me. So about 5:30 a.m. I got awake seeing Don at the foot of the bed gently arranging covers for me and I began to breathe very heavily. It felt like a huge weight on my chest. I tried to lift it off but I realized I couldn't take it off, so for the next half hour I was gasping for breath, and Don was trying to relax me.... I was getting hysterical....poor Don didn't know what to do.....I knew I was dying...." Help me, God. I wanna go home, please....I can't keep on like this." Don tried to give me "Roxy" but I didn't want it....I just wanted to die...."I want to go home," I kept pleading....
    Then I heard Don crying and I tried to mumble the Twenty-Third Psalm....I squeezed his hand tight at "Yea, though I walk through the valley of the shadow of death, I will fear no evil"....It was the end.... I felt so grateful and even though I didn't die, it was what I told Don "a dry run" of what it's supposed to be. By the way, I realize that I'm sometimes a little disoriented with all this dope in me and may be repeating myself. Thank God for dope.
    When I think of how some of my other relatives suffered such pain as they were dying, I'm grateful, but

I'm not dead yet. This is weird. Another "dry run" this morning. That sure is no fun. Trying to catch my breath for ten to fifteen minutes. We're trying to figure out how to handle the moment I get awake till the next ten or fifteen minutes. Any ideas for the next person going through this? Maybe Don has to get me up in the middle of the night and not such an abrupt awakening. Our nurse has helped in giving instructions, but she said each patient responds differently.

Wow! Things are happening around here. Co drops in and keeps us up to date on what she's doing in the house in preparing for this busy weekend with my parents and family here. I can still play cards. What a strange life, if that's what you call it. Have I told you about the choir of angels I hear now and then? It is simply amazing, but I hear celestial voices, perfectly beautiful music coming to my ears. Don wanted to hear them, too, but it's just reserved for me. Also, I hear loud firecrackers now and then, too.

Such wonderful letters and phone calls from so many friends. Thank you, Lord, for all this fun and attention. My last stint here on earth. It is truly fun. I must have dozed off for five hours, 'cause I found Co urging me to get awake; then I go off to sleep again.

Friday, January 7: This is the day my folks are arriving. Look at my condition. Don walked outside the RV with me to see what it would be like to drive ten miles to their hotel in the morning for a big family breakfast. All our kids except Hans will be here, my brother and two sisters, Pop and Mom. But I can't do it. I'm staying in the RV and they'll just have to come to see me. Even with a wheelchair it's impossible to go out anymore.

That was Eunice's last day out of the RV. The family gathered as planned at the hotel for a brunch and a sharing of tales from early days at home on the Ruth farm. Mom, Pop, John, Roma, Martyne (sister) and husband Conrad, Carolyn (sister), all of our children except Hans who lives in Chicago. Eunice's parents like to talk about the experiences with the family as they were growing up. It was a happy family, patriarchal to be sure, but cared for. God (and Pop)-fearing, not a-typical for Mennonite rearing. Our granddaughter, Stephanie, stayed with Eunice in the RV till we returned to Dean's house for a Saturday of talking, planning, singing, and visiting, their last with Eunice. All of this was recorded on video so Eunice could see it.

After a kiss Don is on his way to the motel to meet everyone for the brunch that I'll have to miss. I simply can't handle it, but I look forward to meeting them afterward.

Later: What a wonderful Saturday. It went just the way we hoped and prayed. I can hear church choir and organ again... "Holy, Holy, Holy..." Lots of times, I'm a bit frightened because I hear gun shots and hammers pounding. John, Roma, Pop, Mom, all my kids, Wetzels, my sister, Carolyn. They took turns coming to the RV to talk singly; and that was OK by me. Then John came with Don and Pop and Mom to say "a few words" to clear the air on their theological "misunderstandings." I know they care for me although Pop couldn't say it. He does not seem able to show personal feelings toward someone.

I took the bull by the horns and blurted out, between gasps of oxygen, "I know you've had questions about my spiritual life, but rest assured that I'm right with God. I appreciate so much that you traveled all this way to see me these last days. And I love you; do you accept me the way I am?" .....a brief silence.....John was a gentle and loving mediator in trying to say the right words to make it easy for this short conversation, but I was waiting to hear from Pop and Mom. What were they going to say?

"Eunice, you know I love you," Mom said. I knew she would respond. "We've prayed a lot for you in these days, and know what you must be going through." She likes to speak for Pop. But I was straining to hear Pop say something conciliatory, some word of love.

"Well, I'm going to let God be the judge," is all he could muster. I really wanted them to hug me and lift me off my feet in joy for my life of loving and giving, but it was not to be.

Now the memory still haunts me...was there something I could have done to bring Eunice and Pop together? I never discussed with Eunice alone my disappointment with Pop's response. She would have so cherished a last-minute word of acceptance and appreciation from her father. The strength of confidence in her own spiritual connection to God was supported by myself and many others in her life and she was at peace.

I'm so happy that my heart is right with God and that Don and I have lived with such a secure feeling that we are part of God's redemptive love. I hope that we've been able to communicate that with my parents.

The day ended with the group in the living room, singing, eating, and visiting. I enjoyed watching the video of the day including Pop playing his favorite magic trick game with Jake. He is so good with kids; maybe that's where I got my love for kids. Of course, I cried and cried with Don, tears of joy, mixed with "I'll never see them again" emotion.

The next day was Sunday. They were due to return to Pennsylvania in the morning so there were last "Good-byes" and much crying. I told Mom I would beat her to Heaven's door and be there waiting for her. I know the trip to see us was one that was necessary for them to bring closure to years of uncertainty or real doubts about my spiritual condition, rather it's my guess the doubts were about my not going to church. Actually I never saw them cry. Mom admits that she doesn't have the answer for that lack of emotion; how unfortunate. I waved out the window of the RV as they disappeared over the hill and I will never see them again in this life. Conrad and Martyne took the Ruth family back to the airport, stopping only along the shores of the Pacific at Carlsbad. This was their first view of the great ocean.

I felt so good about the kids today. They came through for Mama. Thanks, kids. I'm so proud of you, and now you're on your own. Don's completely worn out today. No wonder. Phee and Ken were gems and helped with all the practical things like food for the family and kind words; I love them. They have taken to my family like ducks to water.

During the weekend that Eunice's parents were here, they asked what plans were being made for Eunice's burial. I was fearful I might disappoint them about our decision to donate our bodies to science, cremating the remains, and scattering our ashes to the winds. The practice of cremation has never been popular in the Mennonite Church. But to my surprise, Pop and Mom quickly comforted me by saying that their pastor, whom they trust implicitly, was preparing to do the same with his body. The plan was likewise approved by the other members of the Ruth family. Our children fully supported the idea. Eunice had provided so many rich memories for them and the idea that she wanted to be useful after death was only natural.

In the early 1970's, Eunice and I signed papers donating our bodies to Northwestern University Medical School. When we arrived in California in November, I had intended to inquire with the medical school in San Diego about the procedure for body donation, but by the time I got around to it we were entering the Christmas recess and the hospital administration of that department would not be available for two weeks. I was worried that Eunice may not be able to last that long. I pleaded with the hospital operator. She was very kind and said that normally there is at least a two-week waiting period before they would accept body donations, but in light of my predicament she would process the papers herself. Eunice and I were certain we wanted our bodies to be of some practical use in a medical school. It is a simple philosophical point that we are dust and we all return to dust, which then is part of the universe. How the body becomes dust seems a moot point.

***January 10:** It was Monday. The children gathered with Eunice and me in the RV to discuss the weekend with my family. Everyone thought good things had been accomplished. Eunice was so happy it was over, but also was so thankful her parents had traveled that distance to come to see her. She was now on oxygen round the clock. I had arranged her bed so that she could sit upright and rest comfortably, so whenever we gathered to talk, everyone had to crowd around the RV bed to be heard. Eunice wanted it that way. Dean would have been happy if we wanted to use a room in the house.*

Monday night Eunice rested after her usual dosage of Roxanol. We listened to our audio tape and watched the video of the family weekend. I read to her till she was too tired except to put the finishing touches on her diary....

"I sleep and write....sleep and write...I'm O.K. You're O.K....I'm crossin' Jordan alone...."

Those were Eunice's last written words....

Tuesday morning I could see Eunice was getting considerably weaker. She still wanted the children to spend some time with her, but she didn't want to do the talking, nor did she want any more food. She was essentially bedfast, and I was pri-

marily interested in assuring her that she would have no pain if there is anything I could do about it. Attached to her groshong was the morphine dispenser. The nurse had instructed me how to regulate the flow of morphine and to reprogram it to a higher dosage if I chose to do so; she said there isn't a danger of too much at this point. I was well aware that the greater the flow of morphine into her veins, the less pain she would have and also the sooner she would lose consciousness. I was trying to be brave, and I knew that if I had any questions there were nurses nearby.

Tuesday night Eunice still responded, but she kept her eyes closed most of the time. I stayed near her, talked, prayed, and kept her favorite music on the tape machine. She was at peace but fading rapidly.

January 12: By Wednesday morning the only response I got from her were groans which the nurse told me were not of pain but her only way to speak to me. The nurse came periodically throughout the day and told me this was the initial stage of a coma. When I was alone I wanted to talk with her one more time. She responded to my kisses and tears. I read to her Psalm 23. Then I got an urge to call friends from home to allow her to hear them for the last time. It was almost more than I could bear to watch her as she listened to the voices of Letty, Phyllis, and Esther, and others I can't remember. She responded with groans of appreciation (I hope). There was not much more.....I looked at her absent face and shook with grief as I wiped one tear from her eye...and wondered, now forever, why it appeared.

Thursday came. I bathed her again, rolled her body over and oiled her skin for the last time. By afternoon there was no more groaning in response; she was still breathing slowly and I knew the end was near....Is it possible that the brain died and the heart kept on pumping? Does anyone know these eternal questions that don't really require an answer....My children who could stay were taking turns, holding her hand

and talking to her, quietly in awe of the powerful feelings of life meeting death. I wanted to have constant talking and/or music if possible, for what reason I don't know....just an intuition that maybe she would hear....there is a kind of numbing effect where even tears are dried up.

The night was long....I was even wishing to hear barking dogs, anything but this stifling silence....

My mind was racing...what do I do next?

I struggled to remember my last conversation, but I couldn't; and I cried again...what did I say?...what did she say last?...did she answer me?....what were her last endearing words....It all happened before I knew it, and now it was too late! I panicked for a brief period until I realized it was done.

The ship had weathered every wreck..."the prize she sought was won"....she would soon be safe in the harbor and her spirit would again be free. What does it all mean?

January 14: I stayed with her that Friday, the 14th. At noon Tim, Bryan, and Holly went to town with Colleen for lunch, while I sat by her side, holding her hand and talking, hardly knowing what I was saying; I just wanted to be talking. The only other sound in the RV was the quiet voices of two lovers singing "Bramble and the Rose."

I saw a last, hardly visible, breath, and Eunice had taken leave of the body that for all these years had been such a gift of love.

I burst into tears uncontrollably. She joined the choir of angels at last at 2:20 p.m. on Friday, January 14, 1994. At first I was numb, then panicky, not knowing what to do next...there I was alone....I prayed and cried and held her lifeless hand.... here was this tower of strength and imagination, humiliated by a scarred and ravaged body...her heart had pumped its last... she had sung her last song.

The family members returned from town and we all gathered around the bed, held hands and stumbled through "The Lord is my Shepherd....." one more time.

The Hospice care was helpful in arranging for the body to be picked up by the University Hospital of San Diego. Colleen, Tim, Holly, and Bryan were standing with me as we saw the van arrive. I signed the death certificate and then stood aside and watched in shocked disbelief as they wrapped her in a body bag and placed her on the stretcher, then lifted her out of the RV and slid her into the van....how degrading it all looked.... it took less than fifteen minutes, and we watched the van disappear around the curve in the driveway, and then no more... I wanted to drive after it, but couldn't make myself, I was in shock. Those that remained gathered together and gazed into space.

Tim mentioned that the sky appeared more brilliant than usual. I knew Eunice was already getting her wings. But in the RV, it was a quiet night, too quiet, much sobbing and praying, to be sure....the bed seemed so empty. I thought of home in Woodstock, that place she had created, our family of friends, our forty-one years of love, our unfulfilled dreams of growing old together, and now our six children and eight grandchildren who want answers....motherless. I tried to center on her new spirit... what is it like? Can she feel the happiness she so deserved and expected? She has gone on to her new adventure.....

And then I sputtered.....

"The Lord is my shepherd. I shall not want.
  But I am in great need. What do you mean?
He makes me lie down in green pastures,
He leads me beside still waters.
He restores my soul.
  I am waiting, but hurry...how is the soul restored?
He leads me in the paths of righteousness for his name's sake.
Yea, though I walk through the valley of the shadow of death,
I will fear no evil.
  I could never get through those lines with Eunice
  without hearing a knowing moan from her, and me
  crying hysterically....

For thou art with me; thy rod and staff comfort me.
  I felt a quieting, but would it last....
Thou preparest a table before me............
Thou annointest my head with oil. My cup runneth over.
  I am relieved remembering the joy she had in receiving
    all those kind cards and letters, and the expectancy
  she had for the new life.
Surely goodness and mercy shall follow me
    all the days of my life
And I shall dwell in the house of the Lord forever.

...and in the California darkness am I imagining hearing a choir of angels, I believe child-angels, singing with a new choir director...."Everybody needs friends"......

"We can't know why the lily has so brief
  a time to bloom in the warmth
  of sunlight's kiss upon its face
Before it folds its fragrance in
  and bids the world Good Night,
To rest its beauty in a gentler place.

But we can know that nothing that is loved
  is ever lost,
And no one who has ever touched a heart
  can really pass away,
Because some beauty lingers on in each memory
  of which they've been a part."

- *Ellen Breneman*

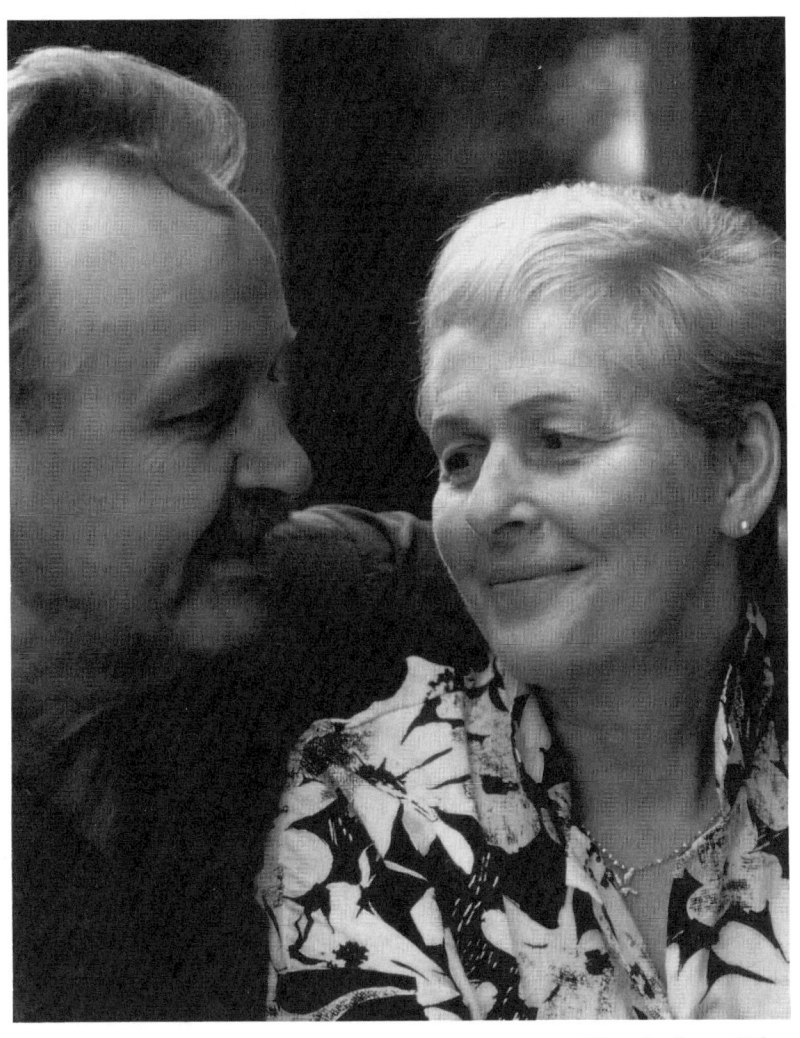

Photo by Susan Urban

Don and Eunice Mast

August 1993

MASTHOUSE

It seems only fitting that all the references about MASTHOUSE SINGALONG made in Eunice's story should be explained briefly, especially because Eunice was the creator of this fifteen-year-old event. It still survives in her memory and welcomes all with open arms the first Saturday night of every month. Banjo picker John McEuen was at our house several times and was so impressed with the place that he called the Chicago Tribune *and persuaded them to send a reporter to write an article. The following appeared in the paper November 28, 1990, written by Hugh Hart, entitled "Stuff of Life."*

Stuff of Life

What may well be the Old Stuff Center of the universe can be found northwest of Chicago in Woodstock, just a few blocks from the town square. The simple white clapboard front of the house doesn't look like much, but once inside, visitors to the home of Don and Eunice Mast are treated to an enormous treasure trove of antiques, art, and bric-a-brac from an earlier era.

In the living room six original Currier and Ives prints that the couple received free from a doctor hang on one wall. In front of a 1910 couch, reupholstered in exchange for lessons by one of Eunice's guitar students, sits an old wagon wheel fitted with a glass top coffee table that they bought at a garage sale. The kitchen massive oak cupboards hold stacks of '40s era Fiesta ware. A set of seventeen frying pans hangs from the ceiling where an ivory keyboard of a dismantled piano has been nailed. Shelved against floor-to-ceiling glass windows are nearly 200 blue, green, golden and clear glass bottles, gleaming in the afternoon sun.

Before ushering their visitors through the eye-popping violet, yellow, royal blue, and green hanging quilt that separates the original house from the Great Room annex, Don, wearing a carpenter's apron, and Eunice, who's whipping up an order of crab quesadilla on a countertop stove bought for $15.00 at a sale, talk about what they proudly describe as the "house that junk built."

"We're scroungers basically. We take what nobody else wants," Don says. "We started pulling stuff out of alleys when we were in college. We had three children and no money. We didn't know much about antiques. Still don't. We just like junk. So between that and having not much cash, the house has just evolved."

The cozy Mast home reflects, in a way no interior designer or slick magazine could, the couple's gradually evolving philosophy that incorporates Pennsylvania Dutch frugality, community activism, and environmental awareness.

The hardwood dance floor in the music room was salvaged from the local high school gym, after suffering water damage. All carpeting was donated or deposited on street curbs. Three restaurant booths in the basement were removed from a local eatery when it went out of business. The vaulted ceiling is anchored by an arch that once was part of the Congregational Church of Walworth, Wisconsin. The arch somehow wound up in a collapsed barn the Masts came across following the Blizzard of '79.

Centerpiece of the addition is the room where up to 150 music lovers gather on the first Saturday of each month for one of Eunice's folk music singalongs. Signatures from the Kingston Trio, Vassar Clements, Taj Mahal,

John McEuen, Pete and Peggy Seeger, and other visitors decorate the wood beams.

Two church pews, bought for $5.00, face the central performing area. Hanging on one wall are guitars, concertinas, bagpipes, balalaikas, banjos, and accordions, mostly donated by neighbors who were clearing out their attics or basements.

The back room of the house is dizzy with knickknacks. Player piano rolls, *Life* magazines from the 1930s, and old doll collections are displayed in a cupboard. Masts' attempt at stained glass work are a pair of "distilfink" birds, representative of early American Mennonite culture, sparkle with the afternoon sun that streams in through the solar designed southern windows. Lying around is a spinning wheel, bonnets, and old plows.

Connecting two portions of the second floor is a swing bridge Don made by roping together the staves of two barrels that were falling apart. "A true Mennonite would cringe at all this; it's hardly spare but, in a way, there is a lavish simplicity to the way it all adds up," Don says.

The southern exposure overlooks an acre of charmingly unkempt pastureland on which stand two guest houses. These were also free, having once been used as Santa's workshop in Woodstock. When the shacks fell victim to vandals, Don pointed out the state of disrepair to local authorities who said, "You can have it if you get it out of here fast."

Other bargains that Eunice found are three brass beds bought for twenty-five cents, and a stunning turn-of-the century sideboard bought by her mother at an auction when Eunice was only ten, for one dime. The Masts imbue their home with a strong community ethic.

Eunice concludes the tour by adding, "We could probably be happy traveling, but we find it rewarding to have a place where people can talk to each other. The way we see it, this house kind of belongs to the community. I guess we're still what you'd call peaceniks, and though we don't go to an organized church, we kind of have the sacred and the secular mixed up in our minds. To us, church is wherever we meet with people. It involves all of life."

The Home Place
(A song adapted by Dee, Jackie, and Jan)

The windows and rafters and shelves are all filled
    With candles and knick-knacks and such;
And I'm gathering you all with my welcoming love
    In this home where we all share so much.

Who will watch my home place?
    Who will tend my heart's dear space?
Who will fill my empty place
    When I am gone from here?

Light splashes through windows on each smiling face,
    As the crowd gathers once again here.
And the warmth and affection enfold this old place;
    We all feel your presence; you're near.

We will tend your home place,
    We will keep your precious space,
Guided by your love and grace,
    We will carry on,
We will tend your home place,
    We will carry on.

Letters From Friends

Phee Sherline from Fallbrook, California, writes... "Ken and I bought our house from Dean Mast, a broker who now lives in Carlsbad, California. As we described to him why we needed lots of parking and a big living room, he said, 'Say no more. You've got to meet my parents.' Ken and I host music parties and house concerts fairly regularly, but we don't even come close to the Mast's. They added a huge room with loft and basement for the purpose. It is filled with chairs, sofas, tables, stuff, all lovingly arranged to welcome the visitor and surprise the eye. It is dedicated to music and fun with practical jokes at every turn. Eunice is a magnificent cook. What is displayed on the bar at the entrance? Fake food! In a house so welcoming, climbers to the loft are greeted by a plaster cobra all but hissing. In surprise, they turn around to find a plaster panther poised to attack from the rear. Collections of dolls, cherubim, teddy bears, dinosaurs, glassware, you name it, are carefully grouped for display. Their home is a riot of joy, color, and activity without three square inches bereft of detail. The joyous atmosphere they create is generously rewarded as musicians from far and near come and play to an audience of 100+. We were seduced. We stayed several days...."

And then Phee touchingly adds some words of a song by Emmy Lou Harris:

> ...I feel a touch, Now will I hold on.
> I see a light, Now will I follow.
> I hear a call, Now will I answer.

"Eunice is that touch, the light, and the call, and we will do our best to answer."

- Phee Sherline

John Hackman writes... "My relationship with Eunice goes back to elementary school in Franconia, Pennsylvania. When Esther and I were married and moved to Evanston, Illinois, in 1968 we met Eunice and Don at Reba Place Fellowship as we too were in search of communal integrity. In 1973, when we moved to Woodstock, Illinois, we renewed our friendship with the Masts.

"Our common heritage as Mennonites, our common paths from Reba Place to Woodstock, our September 1988 trip with the Masts on the Volga River Peace Cruise brought us together in a unique way. And today my relationship with Don and to Eunice spiritually continues to grow.

"Music and people were at the heart of Eunice's life. Love was the highest value. 'Music Alone Shall Live' became the motto of the Masthouse, carved on an oaken sign over the stage. Rather than composing new songs, she breathed new life into the old ones and taught hundreds of people to discover their voices and to find an instrument upon which to join the celebration of life. This reincarnation of the commonplace, the folkplace, still gives hope to many who carry on the tradition of finding community in the common values of common folk."
- *John and Esther Hackman*

"Eunice was the open door with welcoming arms to everyone... so very often to those whom others might shut out. She gave a feeling of being special to those who had no self-confidence, worth, or love. She nourished the dried up seeds of personhood and brought them into bloom. She was the sunlight and nourishing love for those who were perishing from their needs. How many hundreds of times did the two of you watch with pride and joy as someone stepped out on their own for the first time on the stage of the Singalong. She was a walking example of unconditional acceptance and love for so many who could have found it no other way. I mourn for all of us in her absence. One of the greatest tributes we can give to her is to be more loving and affirming to those in need around us in this world so hungry for love. She was a special 'sister' to me in all the right ways. In one of our last conversations she asked about her own worth in God's eyes. It is an interesting phenomena that the purest souls are always concerned about those things...and Eunice was one of the purest, most transparent spirits I've ever known. God is so very much more than the boundaries and names we put on him. You'd think we would finally learn that."
- *Odette Musial*

"It was odd, standing in your kitchen where it blends into the dining room. I found myself gazing at the sticker price on the wall clock. I became lost in memory of different days and evenings years ago when I had begun to know you. It was those dinner parties; not one in particular but the memory of special joyful times, in that very room, undoubtedly, under that very clock that's now for sale along with thousands of other storied memories, the dismantling of a wonderful era in my life. Jan Marsh came by and asked if I was all right and I returned from reverie. You looked well as ever, Eunice. When I saw the sale sign at Rts. 47 and 14 and recognized the address my heart sank, and I felt a bit older. I remember the first time I came to a Singalong here and felt the warmth, the genuine abounding love that emitted from you, and your power with music. I remembered the story of King Saul asking David to play his harp to drive away the demons, to soothe his mind. I think that I would not be exaggerating to say that many who come to that music experience find peace and comfort and love.

"As I look back now to those earlier times when I knew you, they were years of healing, of growing, of developing a higher esteem. When good decent people invite you to sup with them and with their friends, it makes one suspect he may have worth after all; and the suspicions were reinforced time and again. Thank you for sharing your lives."

- Dave Hellenga

"Dear Tom Chapin,

"Thank you for your song, 'Together Tomorrow.' Several years ago I began taking guitar lessons from a wonderful woman, Eunice. One song she taught me was this song. Eunice loved to share her gift of music, no matter if you were a gifted student or just a novice like myself. She always praised and encouraged. And no matter how badly you played, you were always invited and welcomed to perform during the open stage at their monthly singalongs.

"A year or so passed until the announcement of Eunice's diagnosis of cancer. In September 1993 there was a special celebration of music in her honor. It was Eunice's night. I knew what I had to do; I signed myself up for your song. I wanted to show my mentor that I could really do it. I practiced for weeks. Then the big night came. Me and my six-string Sigma alone on stage in front of greater than 250 people in this Masthouse in its eclectic grandeur. I said a few words about how Eunice had taught me the chords to this dreamy song and how the words really ring true. Then I said 'Good-bye' to Eunice and began to cry. Eunice got up from her seat in the audience and stood next to me on stage and softly said, 'You can do it.' So, with her hand on my shoulder, I began to play 'Together Tomorrow.' She joined in with me and sang harmony. It was not the best rendition of the song that the world has ever heard, but it was mine and it was so special to me to be able to pay tribute and show thanks to her by playing and singing with her. Eunice died four months later. Thank you, Tom Chapin."

- Stacy Lasky

"Sacred moments
They are created and they disappear
A thousand times a day, a thousand places.
This place, this church of the Masts
Where more often these sacred moments occur,
A place where God so reliably appears.
Is this heaven? Thank you, Eunice, for your gift
Of soul-quenching!" — *Rosie and Bob Roberts*

"Thank you, Eunice, for sharing your love at the Singalongs. There have been times during those evenings that I have felt closer to God than at anytime ever in church. At those times I've thought, 'Is this what heaven must be like?'"

— *Mike and Ginny Buhrman*

"'Be filled with the spirit, speaking to one another in Psalms and hymns and spiritual songs, singing and making music in your hearts with thanksgiving.' It seems to me like a description of Eunice. She was so radiant with spirit...one of those rare people who seem to have been gifted with a shining spirit and somehow it never got dulled or sullied by the muck of life, or perhaps she was better than most of us at keeping it washed and shined. It doesn't seem real to speak of Eunice in the past...in fact, it isn't real! I am struck at how many lives have been touched by her, and in such a profound way, simply by Eunice being herself." — *Hilda Carper*

"Eunice was truly one of the great people of the earth."
— *Pete Seeger*

"'God be in my head, and in my understanding;
God be in mine eyes, and in my looking;
God be in my mouth, and in my speaking;
God be in my heart, and in my thinking;
God be at mine end, and at my departing.'

"God was at Eunice's end and at her departing. She loved living, and she loved loving her family and friends and wanted like everything to go on living and loving. But she had come to the point of being ready to go; she came to speak of dying as another adventure to go on, 'And you know how I like new adventures,' she said.

"In her last visit with her sister, Martyne, she said softly, 'I'm happy; I'm ready to go. I'm tired of fighting for each breath; I'm at peace.'....the free sharing by the family was largely enabled by Eunice's positive attitude and her openness to share about the departure that was to take place. Eunice, who had enjoyed so much in life and had given so much of herself, still would have had so very much to enjoy and to give, and we who had enjoyed so much with her and received so much from her have undergone a very great loss indeed.

"Vachel Lindsay wrote about General Booth entering heaven:
'Booth led boldly with his bass drum,
The saints smiled gravely and they said, 'He's come.'
Jesus came from out the court-house door,
Stretched his hands above the passing poor
Then, in an instant all that blear review
Marched on spotless, clad in raiment new;
The hosts were sandalled, and their wings were fire,
But their noise played havoc with the angel-choir.'

"I have a similar picture of the excitement that was stirring in Heaven a week ago Friday with the news that Eunice was coming. The word was sent through all of Heaven for everyone to come gather round, and to bring their harps if they wanted to, but especially to bring:
The guitars and the recorders,
The autoharps and fiddles and dulcimers,
The banjos and the balalaikas

"For all to take part in a great welcoming Singalong for Eunice! A grand Singalong that has not, I'm sure, played havoc with the angel choir, but has enriched it with color and warmth. Eunice has inherited what was prepared for her."   *- Conrad Wetzel*

"...Eunice, although you are sick, I prefer to think of the remaining days of your vibrant life than of death. You have been dearly loved...your hospitality, cheerfulness, readiness for risk and adventure and faith in God have been a 'boost' to all of us. Dying is part of living, a very important stage in life."   *- John and Louise Miller*

"My dear son Sean (age 4)...how can I tell you about Eunice dying when you loved her so much. You always got so excited when you knew she was coming because she would always bring you some 'snoopy' or some other precious gift. I want to write these memories of Eunice for you so that you will always remember her. We heard about the Masts and their Singalong at a folk gathering in Woodstock. We decided to go figuring there would be 10 or 12 people gathered around a piano singing.

"Wow! Were we wrong. It was different than any coffee house I had ever seen. There was a feeling, a fellowship, surprises and an acceptance of everyone's attempts on the stage regardless of talent. And Eunice was an entertainer bar none. I remember the first time we were invited to their house for supper. I was overwhelmed and terrified to return the invitation because how could I compete with that! Each course was served beautifully and uniquely in a different spot in the house. After hors d'oeuvres in the living room and soup at the round table in the music room, we moved to another corner where we had a music and game break (blockhead) while Eunice fixed a salad at the table. Dinner was in the dining room. We began by singing '606', a Mennonite hymn. Eunice then began the first course by pouring this mush-like stuff on a marble slab in the middle of the table, always homemade bread, and Don serving wine from a bottle with a 3-foot neck. At the end of the evening we had dessert in front of the fireplace, a flaming jubilee of some sort. Eunice delighted in putting very different people together for her parties, something I'd be afraid to do, but it always worked wonderfully.

"The whole evening was unforgettable. How does she do it? We were amazed at their busy life...hundreds of people dropping by their house all month, or invitations to breakfast, lunch, and dinner the same day with different friends. Eunice never spoke unkindly of anyone, always trying to give a reason for a person acting that way.

"Much of their penchant for hard work, order, getting things done comes from their Mennonite background probably, but they always had a mind of their own. They had the courage to turn down Don's family farm to make a life of their own, lived in a commune for 15 years, and started over again at 40 with six kids and no savings... and then came the 'magic house' where everyone now enjoys the Singalong, the 'house that junque built' as they say. Eunice is an avid garage-sale goer, but she has a wonderful knack for putting it all together in the craziest places and making it wonderful. As many times as we'd been in that house, we could still always find something we hadn't noticed before.

"You're thinking she must have some bad qualities; nobody can be that good. HMMMM. Well, she can be strong-willed, stubborn, but she puts these to good use. Eunice would say that 'pride' is her sin. But why not? Look at the results.

"But now I want to tell you about the dearest memories I have of Eunice. She loved you! Even before you were born, she let me be excited about you, more than any other person, she helped me hope and dream what you'd be like. She planned an entire Singalong around my 'surprise.'

"I've learned so much about giving joy, helping others find joy in songs, games, and being silly. I learned it from Eunice. She taught me to love bubbles. When I'm singing to kids, I often pull a 'Eunice' out of my hat. She taught guitar in a way that people loved music, not just the technical terms.

"I'd always thought some miracle would come along that would pull Eunice through. Steve and I often sing, 'The day of the Clipper' and at the last line: 'The masts will rise again,' I keep hoping I will see her, but things don't happen that way, Sean. Eunice is getting tired now, and she can't fight cancer much longer. Selfishly, we all want her to hang on, but God must want her more, darlin'. There's got to be some serious shaking up of that 'angel choir' up there with Eunice's arriving. There's still so much I want to tell her...'Aunt' Eunice loved you."

- Sylvia Francois

"Dear Eunice...I anguish at the thought of you in pain ...and then when I told you my predicament, I got scared to think of you two and felt ashamed for my cowardice. The beauty of what you represent lies in the fact that neither of you really know what you did for all the places you've been, nor were you trying to be that prominent an influence. As I began to consider a way to grasp the effect you have on me or especially the community around Woodstock, I looked for a way to quantify it. I looked for a way to help you...good family surrounding you, love emanating from around the world literally), the peace in knowing your life has been rich and full of good things....all these you have; so what can I give (in the spirit of the little drummer boy)....your unequivocal support of those less fortunate than you... Eunice, I think of all the songs you taught me; they will be in my heart forever. I love you more than I can write. Eunice, I want to play in your band in the hereafter. Don't worry though, I'll bring my own guitar. Remember, it's o.k. to be scared, to hurt, and to let others grieve...."

- Alex Roberts

"...I feel like Mom is still right here with me. She's such a strong spirit that her presence in my mind and heart is still very real. I do, however, miss being able to just pick up the phone and talk to her about life and all the people and things she involved herself in, and I feel sad when I'm seeing or doing something I know she would love. She was and is an inspiration to live life fully and joyously and when it's time, we need to let go with faith in a loving God and a willingness and wonderment for the 'next adventure.' I know many of us learned how to accept life on life's terms a little better from seeing her doing it so well...what a woman! What a Mom! What a friend! She really loved life and did it so well.

"She seems like a dream, one moment here, so real and tangible, the next a quiet memory. Her physical death is a reminder to me that all things are temporary and to give it all you got while you're here, be happy and help others in whatever way you can while doing the right things for your own self-growth.

"I wear a guardian angel pin from Mom's jewelry box, and I think of her as my guardian angel now. Whenever I want guidance or need serenity, I think of her, pray to the spirit of love that connects us all—God, let go of whatever I'm stressing out about, and know everything is exactly all right. All I have to do is put out a little more love and acceptance. Hey, it works...o.k.?"

- Letter from Colleen

"....we will never forget Eunice, how she has influenced the course of our lives, by enormously enlarging our horizons with friendships and music and in its path we now have a house full of musicians. Our children's interest in music started with Eunice and we have promised to extend that joy to others...."

- Jeff and Avis Fisher

"...I share in the loss of Eunice. Beyond the boundaries of time I see the two brightest stars still spreading their brilliant light over the darkness. The light that you have created and shared and enjoyed over a lifetime will never be dimmed. Because of that I can embrace you in my heart and forgive my tears and sing, in triumphant voice.... Rejoice!"

- Rebecca Strong

"...always in motion, hands busy, smells of yeast, humming a tune, practicing while working for the evening Singalong. Phone rings, she picks it up; the world stops as she gives her attention to the person speaking...then the return to her work, the mending, blow-torching the candles for a neater look, tending her plants, dusting the furniture...she is the maid in this house....coming by a picture of the family and a pause, a prayer; her soul feels rested, her children will make their mark, extending parts of her. She remembered her last words to them, 'Go out into the world and make a difference.'"

- Daughter Jill

"...Don, I want to thank you for making Eunice, Eunice. There could have been no 'Eunice' without your contribution that allowed her to flower and be the best that she could be. Her triumph in music and life and death is in part, yours and I really believe that she is pulling you along this route. I appreciate the ability you have to get people to reach out of themselves and sing. Eunice was like a Merlin to me, and I can't help but think that like Merlin, she is now on another plane, as active and vibrant as ever. It makes me look forward to Heaven and it makes me really value music as ministry."

- Marty McCormack

"...the three-way telephone memorial service between California—Woodstock—and Pennsylvania was a profound experience for all of us who were there. The whole experience was beyond appreciation of Eunice and you, but truly a statement that the greatest thing is love, and that it is possible to live the way of love, and love never ceaseth! And love was so incarnated in Eunice indeed!..."

- Vera Stoehr

"...I have thought of you many times this week. Of how the ministry of music gathered the community around you, of your last hours together and what it must be like to say 'good-bye' to one who is as near to you as your own life, and of you now that Eunice has gone.

"I know that grieving takes a long time. This is because grief is yet another way of loving. Our grief is only as deep as our love. There

are no easy answers. We do not know why a life ends when it does. We do not know why God allows pain.
    "I believe, though, that God does not desert us. God lives with us in the pain. But still that is slim comfort sometimes. The sense of loss, the emptiness, the almost bottomless yearning is too much. But there are friends, and while they cannot take pain away, their love brings not so much comfort as reassurance that love and companionship will eventually, in the future that seems dim, win a victory over sadness. But most of all there is the presence in her very absence of Eunice. There will be moments when her presence will be so vivid, so real. Though there will be pain and sadness in those moments, it will be hard to relinquish them as grief lessens, for as grief passes the intensity of memories fade. When one loves deeply, there is no escape from pain. But there is also the promise of something on the other side of grief."   *- Jim Lehman*

    "...(Eunice's) presence with us will be missed. I'll never forget her joy and love of life, laughter, singing. Mast reunions were always so exciting because of her. My kids remembered the 'lady who played guitar and taught us so many songs, and she even got daddy to wear a pig nose' and she gave cute little gifts to each of them."   *- Marilyn*

    "...I remember Eunice smiling her warm, loving, special smile, and telling me to be sure to come back and sing at the next Singalong. Eunice patting my hand when I was crying after listening to Deirdre Rittenhouse sing 'Velveteen,' and saying to me, 'But you're not shabby. You're beautiful.' I didn't believe it at the time, but it still meant a lot hearing it from her.
    "Eunice making it clear that she was there for me without one bit of judgment or blame when my emotional life fell apart. I love you, Eunice, and I miss you, but you will live forever in each of us...all the hundreds and thousands whom you have touched and changed with your love. There can be no better legacy than that!"   *- Susan Urban*

    "...I didn't see Eunice often, but her beautiful face and her joyful spirit were, and still are, clearly imprinted in my mind's eye and on my soul. Her love was pure, her generosity spontaneous and her face was like the sun. She will continue to be a mentor to me; she was the closest resemblance to God a person could be."   *- Janice*

"...by sharing her home with all who would come, Eunice has made us all a little better, a little more generous, and much, much more aware of what a joy it is to make music together...."   *- Jane*

"The train ride from Chicago to Woodstock on that sunny fall morning in 1993 was one of the longest, most bitter-sweet rides of my life. I'd taken that ride before and it had always whizzed by in the anticipation of seeing Don and Eunice and being enveloped in a world of sharing, love, understanding, laughter, and music. But on this day I was going to say good-bye to Eunice. This was auction day where Eunie was wisely reducing her load by selling off her household wares.

"As I entered the house, prospective buyers were already beginning to gobble up the treasures. I finally found Eunice in the garage where she greeted me with her usual smile and a big hug. Then she said, 'Let's take a walk.' For the next 45 minutes we walked, shared, laughed, cried a little, and said our loving 'till we meet again.'

"As we returned through her garden of flowers, a neighbor girl came running to give Eunice a hug. The five-year-old was admiring the flowers when Eunie asked, 'Which do you like best?' The child pointed to a particularly bright flower that God had put to seed. Eunice reached into her pocket, pulled out a bag, and filled it with seeds. She said, 'Here, have your mommy help you plant these seeds next spring.'

"'Would you help me plant them?' the child asked.

"'Of course I will,' Eunice replied.

"It's now January 1996, and increasingly our children are becoming an endangered species. Oh that we would all take Eunie's lesson to heed the little ones; show them the beauty of the day, and leave them with the promise of beauty in the future."   *- Dorothy Wagner*

The following is a letter from Marina Barchenkova whom we met in Russia as we traveled with Bill Shaw of CROSSCURRENTS. She is now living in the U.S. and working as a translator for Russian businessmen who visit.

"...happy memories; they are like kaleidoscope of bright splashes of color with exquisite design featuring Eunice. My first visit to U.S. was July 1989. As my son and I walked into her house in Woodstock we were mesmerized. Now six years later and after many return visits I still have vivid memories of this wonderful woman. What do I remember?...unconditional love, serving delicious pancakes with home-made rhubarb jam to a dozen guests. She had this incredible skill of magically producing a multi-course meal within minutes and carrying on a conversation at the same time. Eunice introduced me to a garage-sale spree one Saturday morning where she made fantastic purchases which she later turned into precious gifts to many of us....and then in Oct 1993, three months before she died, she was the heart of a celebration at Lakeside, Ohio, where she wore a mask and earnestly read the part of Cinderella with a bunny lisp that sent her audience into fits of hysterical laughter. The next morning I woke up to the sounds of happy giggles and giant soap bubbles floating past my window as I saw Eunice teaching two toddlers to see beauty and have fun."

"Eunice perfected the art of living through the art of giving....'Take the candles home with you. We have plenty more.' Or 'I want to teach you a new song.' Her home was like a beautiful sanctuary, a safe and sacred place where all were welcome without concern for life style, religion, race, age or nationality. And in the midst of all her activities, gourmet meals, and music there never seemed a time when she was too busy to sit with a friend over a cup of coffee, to listen, to give a warm smile, to laugh, and to comfort. During her last months of life Eunie continued to live each day to the fullest, giving far more to others than anyone could return. Her music was wonderful, eyes radiant, spirit captivating. Even amidst rare tears she was not sad for herself. We miss you, Eunie, and we try to live each day a little better because of your spiritual and material nourishment." - *Letter from Bill Shaw*

"I keep a picture of Eunice at my college desk. Whenever I look up, there she is with her glasses set low on her nose, with that look of command in her eyes. Her look helps me keep promises. Don and Eunice form a solid wall against the ugly and the cheap, the whining, the excuses, the urge to give in. The example of their lives obliterates the illusion of powerlessness. Their love was unconditional, their giving all-embracing. I take courage in having them near me." - *Dee Abbate-Winkel*

Chronology of Medical Information

> **November 13, 1987** - First documented visit to Dr. Lesser.
>
> **October 29, 1990** - First documented complaint of problems with left breast (see below).
>
> **July 8, 1991** - Left breast modified radical mastectomy.
>
> **June 1, 1992** - Last documented visit to Dr. Lesser.
>
> **January 14, 1994** - Death

November 13, 1987 - First documented visit to Dr. M. Lesser. Eunice was fifty-four years old at that time and an EKG was taken.

November 24, 1987 - PAP class I (normal) and BP normal.

March 3, 1988 - Routine blood and urine testing showed low hemoglobin and hematocrit; and high cholesterol (handwritten note says "diet").

July 12, 1988 - Mammogram at Memorial Hospital ordered by Lesser. Radiologist: Mark Schiffer, M.D. compared to previous mammograms of 1975, 1985, and 1987, "By history, there is no palpable mass in either breast. There are benign macrocalcifications in the left breast. There is some scattered smaller but benign-appearing calcifications in the lower right breast. No evidence of malignancy."

September 18, 1989 - Pap smear, class I (normal) HDL cholesterol is low. LDL cholesterol is normal. Office visit Pap smear/cholesterol check. Complaints: left knee pain, stiffness, dull pain at night. Labs show anemia.

September 26, 1989 - Blood work (Hgh, RBC, Hct, Iron, and MCH all low; A/G Ratio high); handwritten note states, "anemic."

October 2, 1989 - Ultrasound, pelvis, ordered by Lesser; uterin fibroids diagnosed (in handwritten note), mammogram also taken, ordered by Lesser. Previous mammograms were compared 7/12/88. "Pt. was examined two weeks ago and has no complaints. There are two benign macrocalcifications in the left breast and one in the right. There is no skin thickening or nipple retraction. No evidence of malignancy in either breast." Radiologist: Mark Schiffer, M.D.

November 13, 1989 - Air Contrast Barium Enema. Simple diverticula in upper sigmoid colon. Essentially normal ACBE. Handwritten note "call:normal." Office visit 11/13/89 because feeling week. In fo 'flex.' Started period early, so we are doing the flex because of the anemia evaluation. Plan: patient placed on iron, and Provera. She may need a D & C and/or hysterectomy.

June 5, 1990 - Office visit. Pap smear, mole on right thigh, knee locks when she kneels. Impression: the mole should be removed. Blood work shows low HDL cholesterol and high LDL cholesterol.

July 30, 1990 - Mole on right thigh removed by incision in Lesser's office. Pathology report by J.G. Vega, M.D. states that the mole was benign and completely excised.

August 9, 1990 - Office visit. Sutures from mole incision removed.

September 19, 1990 - Flu shot.

October 9, 1990 - Pap smear is normal.

October 29, 1990 - DISCOLORATION ON LEFT BREAST. "Left breast shows an area of discoloration as described in drawing." Impression: cervical dysplasia & BREAST ABNORMALITY. Plan: Mammograms and colposcopy.

November 20, 1990 - Mammogram. No evidence of malignancy. Radiologist: M. Schiffer, M.D. Looked at prior mammograms, including 10/2/89. No changes. "There is a dense parenchymal pattern in the upper outer portion of each breast...There are two small lymph nodes in the axillary tail of the right breast. There are additional nodes in each axilla. The presence of these lymph nodes is no specific significance. There is no suspicious cluster of microcalcification in either breast. There are two benign macrocalcifications in the left breast, as there were on the old exams."

November 20, 1990 - Colposcopy at Kishwaukee Valley Medical Group, S.C. History: Had a class II pap in September, 1990 and cryosurgery twice by Dr. Felones. Plan: estrogen vaginal cream with follow up pap in 4 months. Finding: "unsatisfactory exam."

November 21, 1990 - Endocervical curettings. No abnormality.

May 14, 1991 - Follow up pap smear for cervical dysplasia. Finding: "cervical dysplasia."

May 15, 1991 - Pap smear.

July 2, 1991 - "In for breast check, the redness has come back and it is more thickened in that area, now the skin has changed." The area of previous discoloration on 10/90 is now gone, there was an area inferior to the nipple now on the left breast there is an area of inflammation above the nipple, there is a peau d'orange appearance to the skin, which is thickening in that area without definitive mass, there are no palpable lymph nodes either in the axilla or in the neck. Impression: abnormal breast exam, possible inflammatory carcinoma versus benign inflammation. Discussed with Dr. Lind. He will see her this week. Will go from there.

July 6, 1991 - S.M.Lesser, M.D. long typewritten history and physical: "This is a 57 year old female who comes in with an abnormal self-breast exam. In October of 1990, she noticed an area of discoloration in the inferior portion of the breast. At that time in the inferior portion of the left breast, there was a slightly reddened area. There were no other breast abnormalities palpa ble at that time and her mammograms were normal. Since that time, she states that discoloration has gone, but now she has discoloration in the upper part of the breast and is thickened in that area. An exam on 7/2/91 reveals a peau d' orange appearance to the skin with thickening in that area, with now inflammation and redness above the nipple. The area that was previously abnormal in 1990 is currently normal. The patient states that the other area did go away and that this area is new. She is not sure of the time that this change has been present. Mammograms have been scheduled and the patient has been seen by Dr. Lind who concurs with our recommendation for breast biopsy to rule out an inflammatory carcinoma versus a benign inflammation. The right breast is normal. The left breast shows an area in the upper part of the breast that shows inflammation, peau d'orange and thickening without appearance of a definite mass. No palpable lymph nodes in the axillae on either side. Plan: Breast biopsy.

July 8, 1991 - Dr. Lind performed surgery: excisional biopsy of left breast lesion & modified radical mastectomy of left breast: "metastatic tumor present in 14 lymph nodes out of 21 lymph nodes dissected." clinical diagnosis: LEFT BREAST MASS WITH ERYTHEMA OF SKIN.

July 8, 1991 - Consultation report by R.E. Lind, M.D. "Patient was recently evaluated in my office at the request of Dr. Lesser for an abnormality of the left breast. Patient states that she has had a strange sensation in the breast for quite sometime. Approximately 7-8 months ago, she developed occasional changes in the left breast. At that time, reportedly, there was no palpable abnormality and a mammogram revealed no evidence of malignancy. After that she continued to have erythematous changes from time to time in the left breast, and now has a palpable mass in the superior aspect of the left breast.

July 8, 1991 - Operative report. Dr. Lind's post-op diagnosis. Invasive ductal carcinoma of the breast.

July 11, 1991 - Mammogram of right breast, normal. CT scan of the chest; routine post-mastectomy CT. Discharge Summary, "final diagnosis: Left breast carcinoma" "follow up with Dr. Lesser in the office. Will be set up for chemotherapy and radiation therapy."

July 23, 1991 - Office visit with Dr. Lesser. "Waiting for second opinion."

August 2, 1991 - Milwaukee County Medical Complex viewed pathology slides for a second opinion. Diagnosis: "1. Infiltrating ductal carcinoma, Grade III/III. 2. 29 lymph nodes, 17 with metastatic ductal carcinoma."

September 9, 1991 - Complaining of brown, melodorous vaginal discharge, impression: vaginitis.

September 20, 1991 - H & P by Lesser for insertion of Groshong catheter for venous access for chemotherapy. Catheter to be inserted by Dr. Lind.

November 15, 1991 - Pap smear, routine check and flex. Complains bright red rectal bleeding, nausea and constipation. Diagnosis: breast cancer. She is almost done with chemotherapy; will repeat her scans following that and go from there.

November 18, 1991 - Pap smear. Abnormal smear. Atypical squamous cells of undetermined significance: dysplasia cannot be ruled out.

December 9, 1991 - Eunice asked why she was here at office (handwritten note, presumably written by nurse). Pap smear discussed, will routine check that in 6 months, set up with radiation therapy arrangements being made.

December 17, 1991 - Blood work; handwritten note says, "Call to Dr. Tanner NML radiation therapy." Blood work was requested as preparation for radiation therapy.

December 18, 1991 - Right mammogram. Compared to 7/11/91 mammogram. No evidence of malignancy. Bone scan. Compared to 7/19/91 bone scan no change. No evidence of metastatic bone disease. CT of abdomen with contrast. No evidence of metastatic disease. Frontal and lateral chest x-ray. Compared to 7/6/91. Normal.
January 6, 1992 - Started on Tamoxifin.
February 4, 1992 - Blood work. "Questionable" lump under left breast. PE area of the previous catheter shows a slight 1cm. lump, minimally tender. The area that she is concerned about is a prominent fold of tissue over a prominent rib on the left, no abnormal masses could be palpated, the axilla were normal. Impression possible low-grade infection catheter site. Plan: put her on Keflex for the catheter site.
April 7, 1992 - "Right breast cyst?" The rest of the handwritten notes are illegible. "Questionable cyst in right breast. At the 6 o'clock position just at the areola there is a 1cm. cystic structure. Aspiration was attempted but failed. Set up for mammogram and ultrasound, have Dr. Lind see her, I do not think that there is any malignancy in this area.
April 13, 1992 - Mammogram right breast. Compared to 12/18/91. No evidence of malignancy. Radiologist: M. Schiffer, M.D. Ultrasound of right breast. Cannot find a cyst at the area palpated by patient. "We must ask the clinician to base judgments as to whether biopsy is necessary, primarily on the follow-up clinical exams."
April 15, 1992 - Dr. Lind's consultation report. 1cm. soft nodular area in the medial aspect of the right breast areola. No overlying skin change. Plan: right breast biopsy and frozen section followed by possible modified radical mastectomy & excision of redundant skin of the left chest wall. No malignancy found in right breast.
May 5, 1992 - Set up for CT scan and bone scan.
May 11, 1992 - Bone scan. No evidence of metastatic disease CT of abdomen with and without contrast. Normal.
June 1, 1992 - Check left breast area. Pap smear. Patient is concerned about the left breast area because it is red and inflamed. There is evidence of inflammation, tenderness, induration and warmth along the entire incision line, there is some fluctuance in one area, aspiration revealed old blood o/w STC. Impression: probable late onset hematoma/cellulitis.
June 2, 1992 - Pap smear normal.

OBITUARY OF EUNICE RUTH MAST

Eunice Ruth Mast, 60, of Woodstock, Illinois, died on Friday, January 14, 1994, at the home of her son Dean Mast in Fallbrook, California.

She was the wife of Donald Clair Mast, originally of Atglen, Pennsylvania, whom she married in the Mast farmhouse in 1952.

Born on a farm in Lower Salford Township, north of Philadelphia, Pennsylvania, in 1933, she was the third child of Henry and Susan Landis Ruth. She graduated from the Lower Salford Elementary School in 1947, and from Eastern Mennonite High School in 1951.

Having been among the founding members of the Reba Place Fellowship in Evanston, Illinois, Mr. and Mrs. Mast moved in 1972 to Woodstock, Illinois, where they have resided since.

In Woodstock Mrs. Mast gave music lessons on a variety of folk instruments, and the Masthouse became the scene of monthly community singalongs for fourteen years. In 1984, '88, and '90 the Masts traveled to the Soviet Union where they performed with other folk artists. The Singalong on September 3, 1993, was held in honor of Mrs. Mast, in recognition of the fact of her advanced cancer. This eight-hour session was videotaped and edited into a program entitled "There was Music."

In addition to her husband, Mrs. Mast is survived by both parents, Henry and Susan Ruth, of the Souderton (Pennsylvania) Mennonite Homes, and the following children: Dean of Carlsbad, Calif.; Colleen, Hawaii; Timothy, San Diego; Jill, San Diego; Peter, San Diego; and Hans of Crystal Lake. In addition to eight grandchildren, she leaves a brother John L. Ruth of Harleysville, Pennsylvania, and sisters: Lois Kennell, Rochester, Minnesota; Martyne Wetzel, Gibson City, Illinois; and Carolyn Ruth, Rancho Cuchamongo, California.

Friends are invited to a joint memorial observance to be held in the Fellowship Hall of the Salford Mennonite Church, Harleysville, Pennsylvania, on Sunday, January 23, 1994, at 4:00 p.m. Sound connection via speaker-telephone will be maintained with simultaneous memorial gatherings at the Masthouse in Woodstock, Illinois (3:00 p.m.) and the Dean Mast home in Fallbrook, California (1:00 p.m.).

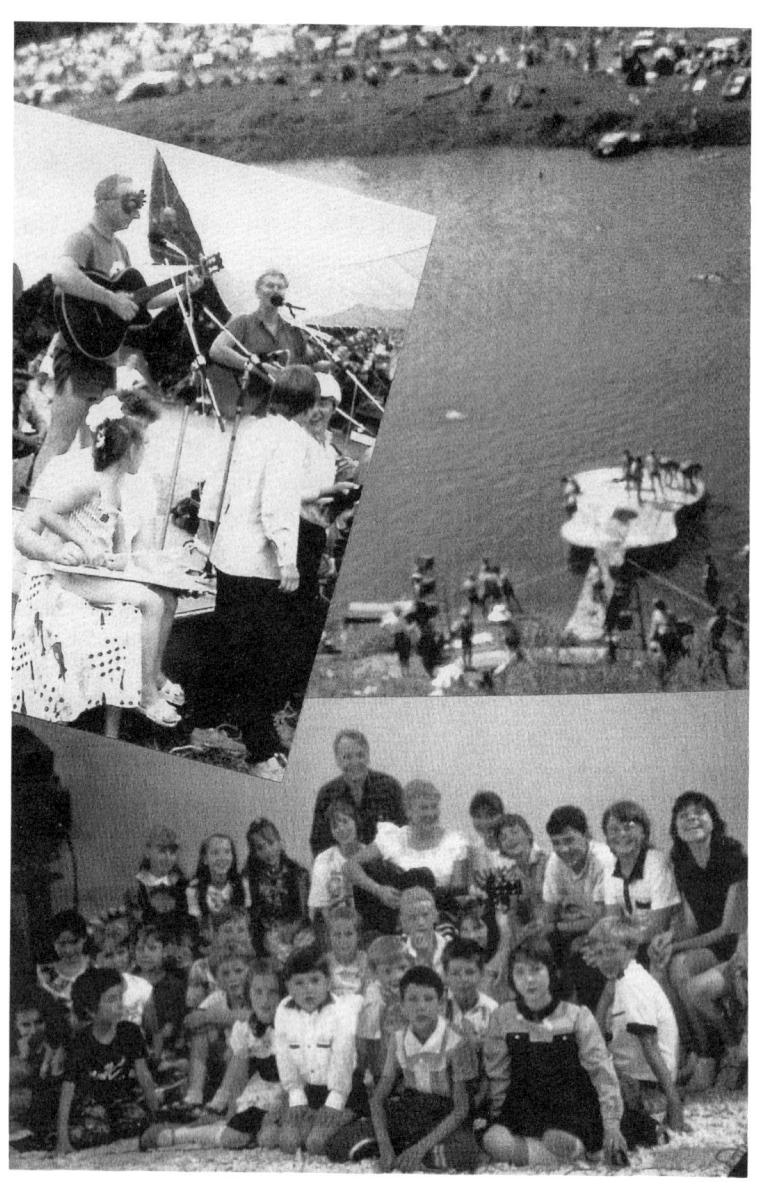

Top: *Guitar stage extends into the Volga River at the 1990 Volga Festival when fifty to seventy thousand persons camped on the opposite bank.* ***Center on left:*** *Eunice and Sergei Nikitin singing Pete Seeger's "Rooster Song" at the 1990 Volga Festival. The other performers are playing a variety of Eunice's instruments.* ***Bottom:*** *Eunice and Don on a 1990 Russian TV program with children.*

The Queen of Love

These lyrics were written and set to music
by Don Mast in memory of Eunice, one week after she died.

Last night I dreamed I saw her face
In some familiar kind of place;
I called her name, she seemed surprised,
Then reached her hand and dried my eyes.
A crowd had gathered close to her;
She touched each one, then slowly turned
And motioned me to come and sing;
We all stood singing in a ring....

"If the people lived their lives as if it were a song,
For singing out of light provides the music for the stars
To be dancing circles in the night."

Her sincere way unmasked us all,
Kingston Trio, the Russians, and Taj Mahal.
We all admired her spontaneous grace,
Like planting a nose on Seeger's face;
Guitars and banjos everywhere,
Songs and laughter filled the air,
Bubbles and puppets, and all those funny songs,
She made each one of us belong.

When I awoke it wasn't real
Groped desperately and tried to feel
Her tender body close to mine,
Just sweet illusions, now I find.....

Lo, she is here, I feel her pass,
The Queen of Love of every class,
Lo, she is here, I feel her pass,
The Queen of Love of every class.

A Singalong Evening

Photo by R. W. Block

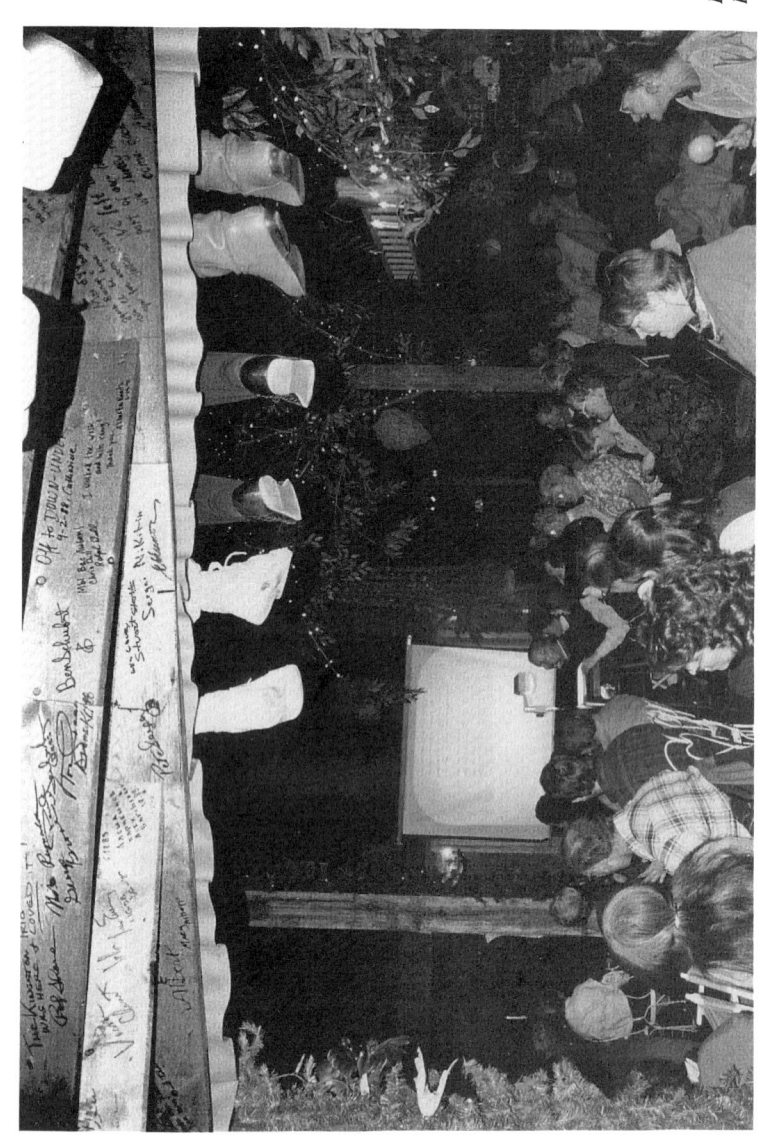

THERE WAS MUSIC

This song by Stuart Stotts became for Eunice and Don a theme song during the last several months that Eunice was alive. Also the words were used for the title of a video in Eunice's memory. Stuart sang the song with Eunice on the video. (Words are adapted by Don Mast.)

Chorus: ...There was music in Eunice's house
There was music all around;
There was music in Eunice's house
And my heart is still full of the sound.

There were wind chimes in the window,
Bells inside the clock,
An organ in the parlor, and tunes in the music box;
She sang while she was cooking or working in the yard;
She sang although her breathing was real hard.

She taught us all guitar, she really had the ear,
She could play an instrument to any tune she'd hear;
I learned so many songs from her
That I love to sing and play;
I guess I will until my dying day.

Those days come back so clearly,
Oh it seems like yesterday;
She gave me so many gifts that I love to give away;
And when she finally died, she sang her last song,
We all sat in the living room singing all night long....

Final Chorus: ...Singing la, la, la (2)
Singin' all those gospel songs,
Singin' all the folk songs;
la, la, la...la, la, la
Singin' all the songs to send her home.

> *do not stand at my grave and weep*
> *i am not there, i do not sleep.*
> *i am a thousand winds that blow*
> *i am the diamond glint on snow*
> *i am the sunlight on ripened grain*
> *i am the gentle autumn rain*
> *when you wake in the morning hush,*
> *i am the swift uplifting rush*
> *of quiet birds in circling flight*
> *i am the soft starlight at night*
> *do not stand at my grave and weep,*
> *i am not there, i do not sleep.*
>   *- american indian*

This was a card that Colleen had found in the fall of 1993 and bought out all that the store had in stock in order to send to family and friends. It seemed so comforting and appropriate now. The day after Eunice died I opened the envelope she had placed in my desk with the instructions: "Open only when I graduate." It was this same card written six months before. She had, of course, written loving farewells to us and all her friends, ending with her encouragement, "Go out and make a difference!"

Don Mast
528 E. Calhoun
Woodstock, IL 60098